Also Available From the American Ac

By Dr Kenneth Ginsbu

For Parents

Building Resilience in Children and Teens: Giving Kids Roots and Wings

Congrats—You're Having a Teen! Strengthen Your Family and Raise a Good Person

For Professionals

Reaching Teens: Strength-Based, Trauma-Sensitive, Resilience-Building
Communication Strategies Rooted in Positive Youth Development

Additional Books for Parents

ADHD: What Every Parent Needs to Know

Autism Spectrum Disorder: What Every Parent Needs to Know

Building Happier Kids: Stress-busting Tools for Parents

Caring for Your School-Age Child: Ages 5–12

Digging Into Nature: Outdoor Adventures for Happier and Healthier Kids

Family Fit Plan: A 30-Day Wellness Transformation

High Five Discipline: Positive Parenting for Happy, Healthy, Well-Behaved Kids

My Child Is Sick! Expert Advice for Managing Common Illnesses and Injuries

Nurturing Boys to Be Better Men: Gender Equality Starts at Home

Parenting Through Puberty: Mood Swings, Acne, and Growing Pains

Quirky Kids: Understanding and Supporting Your Child With
Developmental Differences

Raising an Organized Child: 5 Steps to Boost Independence, Ease Frustration,
and Promote Confidence

You-ology: A Puberty Guide for EVERY Body

To find additional AAP books for parents, visit **aap.org/shopaap-for-parents**,
amazon.com/americanacademyofpediatrics, or your favorite bookseller or library.

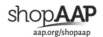

aap.org/shopaap

For more pediatrician-approved advice and the latest updates, visit
HealthyChildren.org, the official AAP website for parents.

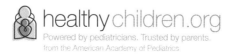

LIGHTHOUSE PARENTING

Raising Your Child With Loving Guidance for a Lifelong Bond

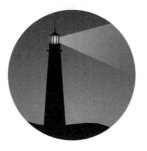

Kenneth R. Ginsburg,
MD, MS Ed, FAAP

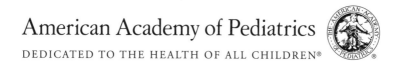

American Academy of Pediatrics

DEDICATED TO THE HEALTH OF ALL CHILDREN®

American Academy of Pediatrics Publishing Staff

Mary Lou White, *Chief Product and Services Officer/SVP, Membership, Marketing, and Publishing*

Mark Grimes, *Vice President, Publishing*

Kathryn Sparks, *Senior Editor, Consumer Publishing*

Grace Klooster, *Editorial Assistant*

Jason Crase, *Senior Manager, Production and Editorial Services*

Shannan Martin, *Production Manager, Consumer Publications*

Soraya Alem, *Digital Production Specialist*

Sara Hoerdeman, *Marketing and Acquisitions Manager, Consumer Products*

Published by the American Academy of Pediatrics

345 Park Blvd

Itasca, IL 60143

Telephone: 630/626-6000

Facsimile: 847/434-8000

www.aap.org

The American Academy of Pediatrics is an organization of 67,000 primary care pediatricians, pediatric medical subspecialists, and pediatric surgical specialists dedicated to the health, safety, and well-being of all infants, children, adolescents, and young adults.

The information contained in this publication should not be used as a substitute for the medical care and advice of your pediatrician. There may be variations in treatment that your pediatrician may recommend based on individual facts and circumstances.

Statements and opinions expressed are those of the authors and not necessarily those of the American Academy of Pediatrics.

Any websites, brand names, products, or manufacturers are mentioned for informational and identification purposes only and do not imply an endorsement by the American Academy of Pediatrics (AAP). The AAP is not responsible for the content of external resources. Information was current at the time of publication.

The publishers have made every effort to trace the copyright holders for borrowed materials. If they have inadvertently overlooked any, they will be pleased to make the necessary arrangements at the first opportunity.

This publication has been developed by the American Academy of Pediatrics. The contributors are expert authorities in the field of pediatrics. No commercial involvement of any kind has been solicited or accepted in the development of the content of this publication. Disclosures: The author and contributors report no conflicts of interest.

Every effort is made to keep *Lighthouse Parenting* consistent with the most recent advice and information available from the American Academy of Pediatrics.

Special discounts are available for bulk purchases of this publication. Email Special Sales at nationalaccounts@aap.org for more information.

Printed in the United States of America

9-507/0225   1 2 3 4 5 6 7 8 9 10

CB0136

ISBN: 978-1-61002-719-9

eBook: 978-1-61002-721-2

EPUB: 978-1-61002-720-5

Cover and publication design by Scott Rattray Design

Library of Congress Control Number: 2023941023

What People Are Saying About *Lighthouse Parenting*

Dr Ginsburg's *Lighthouse Parenting* is an antidote to toxic achievement culture. His guidance, backed by extensive research, will help parents and children navigate the pressures of modern-day childhood and adolescence and emerge with a strong, lifelong bond based on who they are, not what they accomplish.

> Jennifer Wallace, author of the *New York Times* bestseller *Never Enough: When Achievement Culture Becomes Toxic—and What We Can Do About It*

There are thousands of parenting books, but this one is in a class of its own. Dr Ken Ginsburg has created a lasting concept—lighthouse parenting—that builds on very solid child development research. In addition, he is with us every step of the way, like the trusted pediatrician he is, offering practical guidance, insight, and caring support. *Lighthouse Parenting* is a real winner!

> Ellen Galinsky, author, *The Breakthrough Years* and *Mind in the Making;* president, Families and Work Institute; and senior research advisor, AASA, the School Superintendents Association

Once again, Dr Kenneth Ginsburg has written a book that seamlessly integrates the best of medical knowledge and the science of human development with wisdom and compassion. *Lighthouse Parenting* constitutes a unique and invaluable resource that both nurtures and inspires parents and teens.

> Richard M. Lerner, PhD, professor, Bergstrom Chair in Applied Developmental Science, and director, Institute for Applied Research in Youth Development, Tufts University

Dr Ginsburg's use of the metaphor of parents as lighthouses offers a compassionate and insightful perspective on how parents can guide their children toward success while maintaining a deep, loving connection. This book provides a wealth of practical strategies not just to help families survive the teenage years but to truly celebrate them. Smartly written and highly accessible, I strongly recommend this book to any parent seeking to nurture resilience and joy in their relationship with their children.

> Wendy Grolnick, PhD, professor of psychology at Clark University and coauthor of *Pressured Parents, Stressed-Out*

Kids: Dealing with Competition While Raising a Successful Child
and *Motivation Myth Busters: Science-Based Strategies to Boost
Motivation in Yourself and Others*

Lighthouse Parenting is a practical, evidence-based guide to raising children, particularly during the vulnerable tween years. Equal parts reassuring, inspiring, and empowering, this indispensable book provides caregivers with all the tools they need to build and sustain a strong relationship with their child—both now and well into adulthood.

> Phyllis L. Fagell, licensed therapist, school counselor, and author
> of *Middle School Matters: The 10 Key Skills Kids Need to Thrive in
> Middle School and Beyond—and How Parents Can Help* and *Middle
> School Superpowers: Raising Resilient Tweens in Turbulent Times*

Ken continues to share meaningful and constructive advice in parenting in yet one more fabulous book. This book is especially needed now when parents are exhausted and facing big questions about where the pandemic left our children socially and what the exact impact social media is having on their mental health. Ken reminds us of the importance of communication in building our relationships with our kids for life. He offers clear and concrete strategies to build those key relationships and to help us support our children as they navigate development and challenges in life.

> Amy Alamar, EdD, author and educator

This book is dedicated to the life and legacy of Dr Ben Deratzou.
Some of us are given an easy template to follow; we simply replicate how we were parented. For others, that template is not as easy to follow. In that case, one can choose to not make parenting a focus of their life or become deeply intentional about getting it right.

Ben was a deeply intentional parent.
He loved his boys with all of his soul. As one of my closest friends, we had many conversations about striking the balance between loving your child without condition while striving to hold them to attainable high expectations.

Author Note

The term "parent" refers to anyone that fulfills the role of primary caregiver for a child. It is understood that children come from a variety of homes and family structures. Many children are raised by grandparents, siblings, other relatives, and foster parents. The term "family" refers to a group in which one or multiple adult caregivers raise a child or children whether or not they are living in the same home.

Equity, Diversity, and Inclusion Statement

The American Academy of Pediatrics is committed to principles of equity, diversity, and inclusion in its publishing program. Editorial boards, author selections, and author transitions (publication succession plans) are designed to include diverse voices that reflect society as a whole. Editor and author teams are encouraged to actively seek out diverse authors and reviewers at all stages of the editorial process. Publishing staff are committed to promoting equity, diversity, and inclusion in all aspects of publication writing, review, and production.

Contents

Part 4

Protection

Part 5

Resilience and Thriving

Part 6

Preparation

Part 7

Reliability

Acknowledgments

I am genuinely grateful and humbled that the American Academy of Pediatrics (AAP) believes I am worthy of conveying knowledge and skills that will strengthen families. I have been so fortunate to have Kathryn Sparks by my side shepherding every step of *Lighthouse Parenting* with such caring, skill, patience, and humor. She has been my close editorial partner for several books because we have a shared mission to support and strengthen families, so they, in turn, will raise children and teens prepared to thrive. Driven by this mission, she continues to hold me accountable to produce work that is both meaningful and accessible. I look back to the beginning of my partnership with the AAP and remain indebted to Mark Grimes and Carolyn Kolbaba who reached out to me many years ago because they believed that my work would benefit children, teens, and families. Peter Lynch, Jeff Mahony, and Barrett Winston have extended that trust and have challenged me to reach to new audiences and tackle new topics. I am also deeply indebted to Elyce Goldstein and Sara Hoerdeman whose mission focus energizes them to work tirelessly to ensure families find the materials likely to best serve them. We all do better when we rely on others to review our thoughts to ensure they are on point. I am appreciative of my peer pediatricians Jennifer Poon, MD, FAAP; Aisha Mohammed, MD; and Marilyn Augustyn, MD, who reviewed this book and offered their wisdom to me.

I also must celebrate the core team at the Center for Parent and Teen Communication (CPTC) (Jill Baker, PhD; Andrew Pool, PhD; Jacques Louis; Eden Pontz; and Taylor Tropea) for their deep understanding of communication strategies that strengthen families. Their constant presence as supportive colleagues have enabled me to invest the energy in writing this book. Dr Andy Pool has worked closely alongside me to ensure that the information included in this book is supported by research conducted by leading thinkers in positive youth and character development. CPTC is able to strengthen and deepen family connections because we are entrusted and empowered to do so by The Hive at Spring Point; the John Templeton Foundation; the Funders for

Adolescent Science Translation; Kathy Fields, MD; Garry Rayant, DDS; and Sue Bevan Baggott and Steve Baggott, as well as other generous donors.

I am so appreciative of the experts who contributed to portions of this work or reviewed my words to ensure that I offered the most meaningful guidance I could. Dr Veronica Svetaz and Dr Tamera Coyne-Beasley crafted Chapter 18, "Human Connection: The Core Ingredient of Resilience and Thriving," with me. Dr Eric Flake shared his years of expertise in Chapter 13, "Parenting Neurodivergent Children." In many cases, I share the work of some of the thought leaders and developmental scientists who have contributed to our understanding of how to support young people to thrive, including building their character strengths. It is a daunting responsibility to summarize their extensive work in a way that is accurate and actionable. I am grateful to the following people who helped to ensure that I drew from their expertise with the integrity their findings merit: Dr Marvin Berkowitz, Dr Anthony Burrow, Dr Angela Duckworth, Dr Carol Dweck, Dr Susan Engel, Dr Ellen Galinsky, and Dr Eranda Jayawickreme.

I could not possibly name all the leaders in youth development and adolescent health and well-being that have inspired me to take action and informed me on how we might best make a difference in young lives. First, I offer my respect and gratitude to the leaders of the positive youth development and resilience movements who inspired me. Rick Little and his team at the International Youth Foundation first elucidated the importance of the primary ingredients needed for healthy youth development: confidence, competence, character, connection, and contribution. Although I have modified these a bit to include coping and control, they originated and solidified the core ideas. I have been honored to know Richard Lerner, PhD, of Tufts University, who was part of that team and is one of the great developmental psychologists of our time. Dr Lerner has spent decades demonstrating that positive youth development efforts indeed work and that caring is another core trait we must actively nurture through our own demonstrations of caring. I was originally moved to action by the words of Karen Pittman of the Forum for Youth Investment. She called for our nation to understand quite simply that "problem free is not fully prepared."

I have been inspired by the work of SpeakUp!, an organization in the Philadelphia region that brings together young people, their parents/caregivers, and educators in a forum where they respectfully listen and learn from each other. In the safe setting they create, participants shift their perspectives and learn the imperative of sharing their thoughts and feelings and drawing support from one another. Next, I have grown to understand how to foster authentic success from my colleagues at Challenge Success. The work of Denise Pope, PhD, and Madeline Levine, PhD, has been foundational in forming my perspective of what we must do to raise our children truly prepared to lead us into the future. I also must credit Nat Kendall-Taylor, PhD, and his team at Frameworks Institute for reinforcing my drive and building my skills to tell the story about development in a way that empowers parents. Dr Joanna Lee Williams has instilled within me a critical understanding that well-intentioned parenting advice, and even research, can be undermining to people if it doesn't consider the complexity of the lives they must navigate.

I have been blessed to work in regional, national, and international settings to promote resilience. I must highlight, however, the opportunity I have had to work with The Hive at Spring Point, a social impact organization in Philadelphia that champions community-driven change and promotes justice. The Hive at Spring Point funds ecosystems of youth-serving, narrative, and policy-focused organizations that are collectively shifting awareness around the potential of adolescence and promoting strength-based practices in youth development. I am learning from colleagues in each of these organizations how best to engage youth and families in strategies that will help them to thrive. We hope to take all that we are learning to help the people, programs, and systems that touch the lives of young people throughout the nation understand the power of respectful, loving adult relationships in the lives of youth. Joanna Berwind and The Hive at Spring Point are my partners along this journey. None of it would be possible without Joanna's vision for the Hive—to amplify voice, choice, and opportunity for all young people.

I am appreciative of the work that the John Templeton Foundation has done to explore how we can best equip youth to build character strengths. My understanding of how to prepare youth to be their best selves has been deeply enriched by the research they have supported and the network of colleagues they have created.

I thank my professional mentors, Gail B. Slap, MD, and Donald Schwarz, MD, FAAP, who had the experience to guide me, the knowledge to enlighten me, and the passion and love of youth to pass on to me. Above all, they repeatedly demonstrated they cared not just about my academic career but about me. I also thank the best teacher I ever had, Judith Lowenthal, PhD, who inspired me (when I was an adolescent) to grasp the potential in every young person. I also am indebted to my colleagues at the Craig-Dalsimer Division of Adolescent Medicine at the Children's Hospital of Philadelphia for teaching me so much about compassionate care and being uniformly supportive of these efforts. Our division is led by Renata Arrington Sanders, MD, MPH, ScM, who has an indefatigable commitment to supporting youth, families, and communities deserving of our focused attention.

My first mentors and teachers, of course, were my parents, Arnold and Marilyn Ginsburg. I learned much of what I have come to see as good parenting in their home. I was also blessed to learn about the strength of family from my grandmother, Belle Moore, who demonstrated unconditional love better than anyone I have known, except for her daughter Marilyn. I hope that I have passed along in some small measure what I learned from them to my own daughters.

When it comes to parenting, I have lived with my mentor and wife, Celia Pretter. I look at my own young adult children, Ilana and Talia, and marvel at the depth of their compassion and their core goodness. In them, I see the investment of Celia's energy and commitment. From them, I continue to learn every day.

Above all, I thank the young people and their families who have let me into their lives. I have been privileged to witness the strength and resilience of our military-affiliated families through my work with the Military Child Education Coalition. I am consistently awed by the love I have seen in families who have entrusted me to care for their children at Children's Hospital of Philadelphia. I am moved by the resilience of many of my patients, but in particular, the youth of Covenant House Pennsylvania, who serve as a constant reminder of the tenacity, strength, and essential goodness of the human spirit.

I choose to be a Lighthouse Parent. A stable force on the shoreline from which my child can measure themself against. I'll send my signals in a way they will choose to trust. I'll look down at the rocks to be sure they don't crash against them. I'll look into the waves and trust they'll learn to ride them, but I am committed to prepare them to do so. I'll remain a source of light they can seek whenever they need a safe and secure return.

Introduction

Countless parents have asked me, "Dr Ken, how soon should I start preparing for my child's adolescence?" Whether they have a toddler or an 11-year-old, my answer is always the same: "Now, right now!" The parents predictably look at their child and then back at me with a look I'd best describe as terrified. I comfort (and calm) them by reassuring them that getting ready for the teen years is not about preaching do-and-don't scripts to your child. It's about laying the foundation for the kind of relationship in which you'll be welcomed as a guide in their journey toward adulthood.

You matter to your child more than any other force in the world. It is your relationship that will enable you to guide them now, prepare them to navigate adolescence wisely, and launch them into adulthood securely. So, whether you're watching your toddler scamper across the room or waiting for your school-aged child to run in the door after sports practice, now is the time to invest in your relationship. It is the strength of our relationships that gets us through life's curveballs and makes it more likely we'll grow stronger for having weathered challenges together.

I hope this book will be helpful to you now regardless of your child's age. However, I am writing it with an eye toward the 8- to 12-year-old (pre- or early adolescent) child. I've written *Congrats—You're Having a Teen! Strengthen Your Family and Raise a Good Person* to support you in seizing the opportunity the teen years provide to further strengthen your relationship.

There are thousands of books on how to raise children but few that explain that how you raise your child will shape your own life. Your child-rearing years involve a little under 2 decades with your child. Much more time will be spent with them as an adult, with the benefit of lifelong mutual reliance and an abundance of joyful moments. Knowing this, you'll understand that the 2 most important words in the title are "Lifelong Bond"! As the parent of 2 adult daughters, I know that open communication that expresses love and clear guidance pays off in cultivating deep, enduring relationships.

Your family will thrive when your child successfully launches as an independent being and when your adult child who is secure in their independence chooses to be *inter*dependent. Key points to note

- Families where members support, comfort, and guide each other turn to each other to celebrate good times and to gain strength in life's tough moments.
- Families where a member feels controlled rather than supported or protected may splinter because those who feel controlled create distance as a way to maintain their independence.
- Families where emotions are dismissed or where being heard feels like a rarity may visit and enjoy each other's company from time to time but do not learn to rely on each other.

This book is about parenting in a way that will position your influence as most meaningful while your child is growing and that may make it more likely your relationship will strengthen over time. It is about being a lighthouse for your child now, so they will always value your stable and protective presence in their life. It's never too early to start, nor is it too late to make positive changes in your life.

Lighthouse Parenting? Another Approach to Parenting?

It's confusing when it seems that new approaches to parenting come in and out of style with the seasons. To make it harder to sort out, some of these approaches offer opposing approaches. Hover like a tiger mom? Trust like a free-range parent? Battling approaches to parenting generate conversations and earn social media clicks but are baffling to parents seeking guidance on how to effectively parent their children.

Ready for some good news? Lighthouse Parenting is not a new approach to parenting at all. It is the action plan to apply "balanced parenting,"[1] an approach that decades of research and experience has proven offers meaningful benefits for children and teens. Balanced parents express both how much we care about our children and how committed we are to doing what it takes to keep them safe.

---

1. Balanced parenting is generally referred to as "authoritative parenting" in research studies.

This means that even as we insist on rules, our children know that they come from a place of love. Balanced parents know that when we offer our children solid roots, they are more likely to find their wings. This means that our children know we support their growing independence while believing in strong families and lifelong *inter*dependence.

Here's the critical news. Children raised in families that apply balanced parenting have greater academic success, higher levels of emotional well-being, fewer behavioral risks, and reduced emotional distress. These impressive outcomes are likely tied to the fact that families that use a balanced approach to parenting also have the closest, warmest, and most communicative relationships.

Lighthouse Parenting is more than a catchy phrase. It embeds an image in our minds that reminds us how to apply the best of what is known about effective parenting. The research around balanced parenting is convincing. But in this book, you'll learn the strategies to put it into action and the words you might use as you apply its proven principles. In Chapter 9, "Parenting for Optimal Influence," we'll discuss in greater detail what we know about its positive effects in contrast to other parenting styles.[2] Chapter 9 will also cover how to move toward this style of parenting, because striking the right balance is tough for many of us, especially if we were parented differently or other adults who are sharing parenting responsibilities differ in their approach. After all, sometimes balance means reaching common ground with another person who also cares about your child but doesn't agree on how to raise them.

Perhaps the greatest strength of Lighthouse Parenting is that it gives you the skills to meet the needs of your child now, but also recognizes that flexibility and responsiveness to evolving circumstances is key to maintaining balance over time. Lighthouse Parenting can be the foundation of a lifelong relationship because its principles allow you to adapt to meet changing needs. Your child will always rely on your ability to see them in a positive light as a reminder of their potential. Your younger child will need your sharpest attention to protect them. Your adolescent will need you to focus more on preparing them to make their own decisions while always remaining clear-eyed about areas they still need protection from. Your child at every age and far into adulthood will rely on your stability as an ever-present force in their life.

---

2. Parenting style was first explored in the 1960s by Dr Diana Baumrind, a renowned developmental psychologist.

Our Journey

For the sake of our families, I hope that this phrase will start many conversations: "I choose to be a Lighthouse Parent . . ." The journey we'll take together is one that allows us to reflect on the key phrases that describe the kind of parents we choose to be. Each of the 7 parts of this book dives into a key point that unfolds into the full statement of intent about what it means to choose being a Lighthouse Parent.

I choose to be a Lighthouse Parent. A stable force on the shoreline from which my child can measure themself against. I'll send my signals in a way they will choose to trust. I'll look down at the rocks to be sure they don't crash against them. I'll look into the waves and trust they'll learn to ride them, but I am committed to prepare them to do so. I'll remain a source of light they can seek whenever they need a safe and secure return.

Part 1: Stability

I choose to be a Lighthouse Parent . . . A stable force on the shoreline.

It is your stability that offers security to your child as they grow and that ultimately will make them want to stay connected with you after they launch into their own independent lives. With a secure base, children can more safely explore the world and develop to their potential.

Part 2: Modeling and Knowing

I choose to be a Lighthouse Parent . . . from which my child can measure themself against.

We are always being watched by our children to see how to navigate a momentary challenge and to imagine what it might look like to be an adult. But role modeling is not the only way your children use you as a measure. How you see them guides their behavior and forms the self-image they strive to maintain.

Part 3: Communicating

I choose to be a Lighthouse Parent . . . I'll send my signals in a way they will choose to trust.

A child knows what you believe and how you expect them to behave by how you communicate. A child gains their own footing by knowing how deeply you love them and trusting that you want them to grow. A child learns to trust their own emotions when you respect what they feel and to make their own decisions when you listen as they think through their plans.

Part 4: Protection

I choose to be a Lighthouse Parent . . . I'll look down at the rocks to be sure they don't crash against them.

As a parent, you celebrate your child stretching but don't allow them to approach true danger. In fact, until you've determined those things that can do irreparable harm, you won't feel confident letting your child venture into unchartered territory. When we do need to dive in to protect them, our children must know that we do so because we care about them, not because we need to control them.

Part 5: Resilience and Thriving

I choose to be a Lighthouse Parent . . . I'll look into the waves and trust they'll learn to ride them.

Waves can make us lose our footing or lift us up. Resilience at its core is about maintaining your footing even when life becomes turbulent. Our goal is not for our children to be resilient, it is for them to thrive. We can lift our children up by supporting them to build those essential character strengths that contribute to human thriving.

Part 6: Preparation

I choose to be a Lighthouse Parent . . . I am committed to prepare them.

The best way to protect your child is to prepare them to have self-control and wise decision-making skills. You'll want them to develop the skills of self-control and to make wise choices even if they're not the ones that will give them the most pleasure in the moment. Ultimately, you'll want them to be able to judge for themself where they can stretch and when they should keep their distance.

Part 7: Reliability

I choose to be a Lighthouse Parent . . . I'll remain a source of light they can seek whenever they need a safe and secure return.

Our children may pull away from us and make some unwise decisions or even serious mistakes. We can restore our relationships and bring our children back to reconnect with their better and wiser selves when we root our actions in the knowledge of all that is good and right about our children. This gives them an understanding of the kind of relationships—with us and with themselves—that they choose to return to. The last chapter in this book underscores the most critical point: Parenting doesn't end when our children launch from our homes. Our goal for our children is to instill lifelong interdependence and mutual support. These are the type of intergenerational relationships in which humans thrive.

Apply Your Wisdom on This Journey

I hope that you use this book as a starting point to reflect on the kind of parent you want to be and to initiate discussions with other caring adults. Please treat my words as guidelines for you to consider rather than as directives you must follow. There are things I simply do not know about you or your child, and one-size-fits-all parenting can never be right. Critically, this book is about striking the right balance in your child's life between the expressions of your caring and the actions you take to keep your child safe. Only you and other caregivers can understand what safety means in your community and among your child's peers. Only you can tailor my written advice for the nature and temperament of your child. Some children need more protection, while others need encouragement to stretch their wings just a little bit further. Apply your wisdom and experience to any guidance I offer.

Being Human

With thousands of books written on parenting, it is easy to conclude that there must be a right way to do it. This perspective can often leave us feeling badly about ourselves because we all experience parenting moments that don't make us proud, and none of us will raise children without any challenges to navigate.

A better way of looking at it is that only something as complex, critical, and difficult as parenting would merit so much attention from experts.

I have rooted the advice in this book in the decades of research that has explored the benefits of balanced parenting. As the founding director of the Center for Parent and Teen Communication, I am mission driven to help strengthen your family to make it the kind of environment where a child or adolescent will grow to be their best self. But I know that having a child is like having your heart on the outside of your body. There is no way you can care about something as passionately as raising your child well and always have things go as you had planned . . . or wished it would.

You do not need to have all the answers. Supportive parenting is about being attentive to signals, remaining unconditionally caring and unwaveringly present. Supportive parenting is about staying solidly present when your child *does* encounter problems. It is about showing up. You can do that!

And being honest with yourself that parenting is difficult and that wise decisions require thoughtfulness makes you the kind of adult your child can use as a model. Being clear about when you need to course correct after a mistake doesn't make you look foolish, it makes you look human. And *being* human is the secret ingredient to raising a *good* human.

Part 1
Stability

I choose to be a Lighthouse Parent . . . **A stable force on the shoreline.**

CHAPTER 1

Your Family as a Source of Stability, Now and Far Into the Future

Don't you love how children dart down a path, zigzag around the yard, race as fast as their little legs can move, and then suddenly stop short as if their batteries ran out? Why, you ask? They stop to be sure their parents are still watching and once reassured, they will continue their adventure.

As the years pass, our children continue to run, stop, and look back. What changes over time is how fast they run and how far they get before stopping. What they're looking for as they glance back also changes over the years. Young children look to us for reassurance that they are safe. Older children and adolescents still expect us to keep them safe but seek out permission, or even encouragement, to continue to explore. If we encourage growth and exploration during adolescence, our adult children will likely continue to look back for affirmation that they are on the right path.

Being There

When your young child looked back to find you, they didn't assess whether every thought you had was filled with wisdom or every feeling you held was well considered. You being there was enough.

Being a Lighthouse Parent is about forging a secure attachment with our children so they'll see us as a source of stability in their lives. A secure attachment, as originally described by developmental psychologist Mary Ainsworth in the 1960s, gives a child a sense of a "secure base." This concept of a "base" is an apt description of what it means to be a source of stability. In baseball, we tag the base, but the goal is to venture forward, and we celebrate when we return home.

We hope to create a home base where children can learn to stretch their limits and have safe experiences with failure. But success is also dependent on them taking advantage of the opportunities for growth and learning outside of our home. Exploration in the outside world oftentimes sets children up for disappointment, failure, and emotional pain. We offer stability when our children learn they can reliably return home knowing we'll help them process their experiences and be empathetic toward their emotions.

This will be the first time I will state what will feel like a refrain in this book: None of us will always find the perfect words to say when our children are experiencing distress. *Being there is what counts.* There is nothing more protective for a child of any age than the unconditional presence of their parent.

There Is Security in Our Complexity

I would challenge you to consider that the real-world complexity of our home life offers young people a greater sense of stability than an idyllic, but false, notion of perfection. I'm not suggesting children should live and thrive in chaotic environments. Rather, young people feel secure when they know that they are cared for by real people with real-life issues who nonetheless continue to prioritize their needs. Our children seek reliability and attention but do not insist on being our sole focus.

The home without any problems—which does not exist—is not the one where young people will feel the most secure. After all, how could you go to someone with a problem if they don't understand that life is often complicated? Would you feel secure sharing your own anxieties and concerns with someone who was trying to create a picture of a home that was perfect? Wouldn't you be afraid of creating waves or disrupting the idyllic image that is trying to be maintained? Wouldn't your fear of disappointing them override your desire to inform them of your struggles?

I'm not proposing that we aim to create disruptions in our homes just to help our young people feel safer within them. But I am suggesting that we be and stay human. Caring humans. People who know and recognize that when times get tough, we are stronger together. People who know that even if we are furious at the people we love, in challenging times, we will still rely on them because their presence is not conditional. When the rest of the world is throwing us curveballs, the people in our home will always have our back.

Ideally, our home is where people can be themselves. Sometimes because young people feel most safe and secure within our homes, it is within our 4 walls that they express their frustrations the loudest. Precisely because of how deeply our children trust our reliability, they'll safely release their anger with us. Have you ever seen a family without sibling squabbles? Odds are you have not. Despite these conflicts, siblings stick with each other, especially when someone outside the home makes one feel insecure.

We must do the hard but meaningful work on ourselves to remain emotionally available to our children. In Chapter 2, we'll discuss how critical it is that your child knows that you have the emotional bandwidth to lend them stability. Our children, even at the youngest ages, can sense our distress. As they grow older, they'll choose to protect us from the complexities of their lives if they believe we are overburdened. Count this as the first nugget of many in this book to emphasize taking care of yourself—for your own sake and as a strategic act of Lighthouse Parenting.

A Haven Nonetheless

The world is a rapidly changing, and sometimes unpredictable, place. **We cannot control everything outside of our homes, but we can be intentional about creating sanctuaries within our homes.** Taking control where we can is key to remaining resilient. We must speak openly about this with our families and express clearly why we are working to create these havens. Consider sharing the following language with your family members/household:

> The world can feel frightening at times. Therefore, we must make our home a safe haven. Let's choose to be kinder and gentler and more open to our differences. We'll take turns drawing strength from each other in different moments. Let's speak openly about how we care about each other, and do so even when we're most frustrated or angry with one another. We'll talk things through and practice forgiveness in this home. We'll grow stronger because we rely on one another.

Notice that I am not suggesting a safe haven is a place to tuck away or deny or dismiss emotions; rather, it must be a place where heightened emotions are processed in a healthy way. The fact that we work through tension and focus on each other's strengths adds a deeper layer of security to our home. When we do this as our children grow, they will learn that they can have conflict and recover. They will learn that it is often with the people with whom we feel safest that we might express ourselves most fully. But it is ultimately our love for each other that ensures we can respectfully work through those uncomfortable moments.

Families Shouldn't Be on Their Own

Parents are undoubtedly the most important people in their children's lives. But children grow stronger when they have many strong connections with people committed to their development. In truth, families are strengthened by their support systems and communities. So, while this book is about empowering parents and strengthening families, I want to state clearly that you shouldn't need to do it alone. Children should be exposed to extended family, schools filled with caring professionals, and community activities. And parents should draw strength from extended family, from their cultural strengths and spiritual traditions, and from rich community connections. Chief among those connections should be other parents raising children and teens. In the spirit of drawing strength from others and developing shared wisdom, I hope you use this book as a conversation starter with other caring adults.

CHAPTER 2

The First Step to Stability: Finding Your Footing

You won't be able to be a stable force for your child unless the ground is solid under your own feet. This chapter discusses 3 action steps to ensure your own secure footing in your parenting journey.

- Committing to your own health and well-being
- Increasing your comfort in incorporating parenting practices that may feel unfamiliar
- Clarifying your parenting goals

Preparing for Adolescence

Adolescents want to know what parents care about and what is expected from them. They feel secure when your reaction is predictable. They'll share what is on their mind when they know their problems will not overwhelm you.

Shaping Your Lifelong Bond

Your adult child will value a mutually reliant relationship and care about your well-being. They too will share their burdens with you only when they know that you are taking care of yourself and therefore have the reserve to hear about their lives.

Attend to Your Own Needs

Your well-being allows you to be emotionally available for your child. Full stop.

Children demonstrate they care about us from the very early years. How did your preschooler demonstrate their empathy to you? Did they stroke your hair to comfort you? Did they offer you kisses and hugs? (If I looked worried, one of my daughters would get me Band-Aids!) When did they begin asking you why you were worried or seemed sad? Adolescents become particularly sensitive to our emotions. Do not believe false notions that suggest they stop caring about their parents.[1] No matter their age, have you noticed your child's mood reflects yours? Have you sensed they become particularly angelic or disappear from your presence when you are otherwise burdened?

Because our children care about us and sense our moods, they may spare us the details of their lives to protect us. This is even true, and perhaps especially true, when our relationships are close. I don't want you to be perfect or to feign stoicism. But I want you to invest in your own well-being for your own sake and for the sake of your children. Self-care will open your bandwidth and it is then that your child will trust that you can be receptive to their thoughts, feelings, and experiences. I have heard versions of the following statement countless times from adolescents who desperately needed their parents' involvement but hid the details of their lives from them:

> I couldn't tell my mom. She has so many things on her mind. She works so hard and doesn't get paid enough. I think she's already depressed with what's going on with my dad. And she takes care of my grandmother. I'm a mess; the last thing she needs is to deal with my problems.

When I encounter this type of situation, I help the young person grasp that they are not sparing their parent by withholding what is going on in their life. They honor them by including them. Then, I guide the parent to have the "Please don't spare me" conversation.

> I love you and appreciate your sensitivity to what I'm going through. I know you're trying to spare me by handling problems on your own. Please don't

---

1. This was disproven in the 1990s by Ellen Galinsky in *Ask the Children: The Breakthrough Study That Reveals How to Succeed at Work and Parenting*. She found that teens want time with their parents, care about their well-being, and value their guidance.

choose to spare me from what's happening in your life. Sometimes, I question how well I am handling things in the rest of my life. But I know being your parent is the most important thing to me and I want to come through for you. If anything, it'll let me focus on what I care about the most—you. Please know that you honor me when you include me in your life.

We are all works in progress. Our children do not need us to be problem free or entirely set our burdens aside. Instead, they need to know that when you get overwhelmed, you have strategies to manage your problems or release your emotions in a healthy way. This will send them the unspoken but clear message that they can add something to your plate without fearing it will be more than you can handle. In the next chapter, we'll discuss how sharing your calm isn't about being unflappable, it's about preparing our children to learn to achieve balance by being transparent about what we do to maintain ours.

You'll parent best when your child knows you are well enough to be their lighthouse. You'll know your child better because they'll share more. You'll better experience their joys. Because your unburdened self is more sensitive to small waves, you'll more effectively avert crises by catching early subtle shifts in your child's mood. Critically, you'll be the person they'll comfortably come to when they need support.

Self-Care Creates Bandwidth

Self-care is usually presented in modern culture as strategies to escape your real life or soothing ways to manage stress. But we better care for ourselves when we integrate strategies to make our real lives more satisfying and productive. If this book increases your confidence as a parent and positions you to strengthen your family as you raise a child prepared to thrive, diving into this book *is* self-care.

Key Steps to Strengthen Yourself

Prioritize love and friendships. While gaining support and nurturance from others, you will also be modeling how important it is to maintain these significant relationships in our lives.

Prioritize sleep. We manage stress and make better decisions when well rested. The efficiency you'll gain will far outweigh the time you've investing in restorative sleep.

Incorporate exercise into your life. The proven effects of exercise in terms of stress management and improved clarity of thought are undeniable. Use exercise as both a way to maintain your physical and emotional health and to "work it out" when you're experiencing an overload of stress. Even 15 or 20 minutes of movement a day makes a difference.

Incorporate relaxation strategies into your lifestyle. Relaxation isn't about getting away from it all. It is about giving yourself the ability to achieve the balance that allows you to refocus. This can look like reading a book, practicing yoga, listening to music, doing light cooking, or taking a short walk.

Express rather than bottle up your emotions. When we set aside our thoughts and feelings, they fester waiting for an inopportune moment to come pouring out. When you express yourself through talking, writing, praying, or any of the creative arts, less tension builds up.

Recognize when you deserve support and reach for it. Being vulnerable *is* being strong when we notice we are deserving of guidance. There may be a time you'll have to guide your child toward professional support; you'll do so much more effectively when they know you view seeking help as an act of strength, not a sign of weakness.

As you do these things to care for yourself, occasionally talk out loud about what you're doing. You'll achieve 2 goals. First, you'll model that we all need to invest in our emotional and physical health and in feeling connected to others. Second, knowing you are caring for yourself will give your children the confidence to reach out to you because they'll set aside their fears of adding something to your overflowing plate.

Commit to Approach Parenting in a Way That Works for Your Family

At its core, the Lighthouse Parenting strategy is about expressing our love while also being clear about our expectations. It is about letting our children explore new territory—and sometimes fail in the process—always with an eye ultimately to their growth. I am confident that these principles will benefit your family now and far into the future. But I don't assume it is easy for families to course correct if they've been doing things differently.

There are a few challenges people navigate as they consider adding new approaches to their parenting repertoire. I want to address these challenges from the onset because any mixed feelings you experience may come out as inconsistency in your parenting practices and that can limit your ability to offer your child the stability that is at the core of Lighthouse Parenting.

The first challenge is that it's not always easy to express how we feel, be firm when it's not popular, or watch from the sidelines when we want to dive in. Second, someone else may be sharing this parenting journey with you, and they may have a different perspective on the best way to raise children. Because stability as a parent is one of your major goals, it makes a lot of sense to reach a compromise and agree on parenting strategies. You don't want parenting styles to become a pain point in your relationship. Third, you're coming to this topic with your own history of being parented. You may find yourself copying the ways you were raised or rejecting them entirely. Why does this generate conflicting feelings? You may have aspects of your upbringing that you remember fondly, as well as unpleasant childhood memories of how you were parented. Or, you may try different parenting practices than how you were raised but worry that doing so implies your own parents did something wrong.

The Bottom Line: Be self-reflective before stretching into parenting practices you know are good for your child but that don't feel familiar or comfortable to you. This is about you being a source of stability and to get there, you must be confident in the choices you're making. I support you in building your skill sets in applying the best of what we know in effective parenting. It's OK, however, to work through these challenges over the long term and incorporate the particular ideas and strategies into your parenting practices as you see them work for you.

Set the Right Goals

You'll maintain your footing if you know what you really stand for. Being intentional about your parenting goals will help you stay grounded in your core values. On any given day, you might feel like you are running on a treadmill trying to keep up because people imply your every decision has consequences for your children. This overly pressured approach to parenting destabilizes parents who are doing the very best they can. If your child is physically and emotionally safe, adequately nourished, and knows without question that you love them, rest assured that you are on the right path.

If you root your own approach to parenting in goals that are focused on raising a good person who cares for themselves and others, you're less likely to be derailed by daily pressures and confusing messages about what effective parenting is. I offer the following suggested goals; review them until the goals that meet your values and expectations are written on this page. Seriously, get a pen and write your own thoughts and goals alongside mine!

Goal 1: Commit to having open communication within your family. No family gets it all right, but when open communication exists people can share values, shape decisions, talk about emotions, and get through tough times together. Critically, you'll be well positioned to course correct relationship challenges within your family.

Goal 2: Prepare each child to navigate the world independently but to simultaneously know the importance of relying on others. Overly controlling parents raise people who want to gain as much distance as possible. Families where growing independence is valued may more comfortably choose mutual reliance and *inter*dependence.

Goal 3: Raise your child to be well prepared to get a second job. We are highly attentive to our children's grades and scores because we focus so much on the next step after they leave our homes (ie, their first job, college, or the military). But we must not forget to focus on the skills that will take them through life. Young people stay at their first job for approximately 2 years; consider what their second boss will be looking for as they consider hiring them. The second boss will likely ask the first boss about their reliability, their collaborative skills, whether they learned on the job, and how they rebounded from failure.

Goal 4: Commit to raising your child with an eye toward who they will be as a 35-year-old. When you do this, you'll stay focused on developing their character strengths (see Part 5 on thriving) and ensure they build relationships in their lives that will be the foundation of their sense of belonging.

CHAPTER 3

Sharing Your Calm: Co-regulation as the Root of Security and Thoughtfulness

People succeed in life when they can tap into both their emotional strength and their thoughtfulness. Our emotions allow us to feel fully and draw strength from connecting to other people. Our thoughtfulness allows us to consider others' feelings, make wise decisions, and look toward the future. There is a balancing act between feelings and thoughts, because when emotions are amplified, the ability to think is limited. Parents can help children achieve this balance. Our youngest children learn to control their emotional impulses when we teach them how to share, be patient while they wait in line, and understand why they need to eat their vegetables before dessert. We build their emotional intelligence when we teach them the language to express their feelings. Once they understand that the word "angry" expresses the rage they feel inside, they can learn to choose healthier ways to express these angry thoughts instead of throwing things or hitting their playmates.

Even adults can be derailed by something that triggers an emotional response. By drawing from a well-earned set of experiences and coping strategies, most adults can collect their feelings so they can thoughtfully approach a problem in a healthy way. Childhood and adolescence are when we build the skill sets that allow us to self-regulate, but the journey is not always easy.

Your ability to lend your calming presence allows your child to steady their emotional responses and create room for problem-solving. Simply, your stability helps your child build their own.

Preparing for Adolescence

Because the emotional centers of their brains are developing rapidly, adolescents can be highly emotional. Your calm helps them access their thoughtfulness to make the wisest decisions. If you are a source of calm during childhood, your tween and teen will continue to turn to you when they need your steady energy to settle themselves.

Shaping Your Lifelong Bond

Upsetting experiences occur throughout our lifetimes and will always interfere with our ability to think clearly. When you are the person your child knows can get them to a calm, thoughtful state, you will always be that person. If your child learns from you the power of a caring, calming presence, when they are an adult, they may become that person for you.

Important Vocabulary to Know

Although parents help children achieve emotional balance, we don't often use the words that describe what we do and the goals we hold for our children. The following terms set the foundation for understanding these goals:

- We want our child to display **self-control**, the ability to pause or control impulses before thinking or acting.
- We need our children to learn **self-regulation**, the emotional state that underlies whether we can move beyond our impulsive reactions, especially in stressful circumstances. Self-regulated people can attend to a problem, maintain their focus, and then thoughtfully address the task.
- **Dysregulation** describes the unsettled state that interferes with action. In a dysregulated state, we are more reactive, impulsive, angry, or out of control.

- We help our children maintain their emotional calm and thoughtfulness through **co-regulation.** We lend our calming energy to support a person to self-regulate until they can develop and then draw from their existing internal resources and strategies.

We Feel What Others Feel

Emotions are contagious and we can catch both feelings of calm and worry. Even panic. We transmit spoken and unspoken signals to one another rapidly and often unconsciously. These will trigger instincts that affect whether we feel relaxed or unsettled, safe or fearful. In the language of brain science, co-regulation is syncing between one person's emotional center to another person's emotional center. This connection between us is essential to our survival because together we can better respond to danger. Children do not need to experience every danger because they instinctively trust adult vigilance. Emotional syncing is key to thriving because it causes us to connect with one another as we rely on collective experience and earned wisdom. You want your child to "catch" your calm emotions so they can feel safe, think productively, and benefit from the range of feelings that make life worth living.

Your child always looks to you for co-regulation

Humans are wired to draw solace from and create safety with each other. But the reliance a child has on their parents is different than any other human relationship. It is the bedrock of security and forms the essence of what will be a lifelong understanding of what human connection and reliance means.

The bond with our parents teaches what human support can offer and ingrains within us an understanding that one day we will offer such protection to others. Our children look to us from the earliest ages to determine how they should react to discomfort or assess danger. When we jumped into action as their hand approached the stove, they learned that it posed real danger. When a 4-year-old slips and skins their knee, they glance at their parent with a "Should I cry now?" look. If a parent checks every limb for a presumed fracture, a child will likely cry and demand a bandage. But if the parent remains calm, determines there is no injury, and says, "Let's wash that off so you can get back to playing," the child may ask to have the knee quickly cleansed so they can get back into action.

Co-regulation: sharing your calm

Imagine yourself on a plane experiencing sudden turbulence. Your stomach sinks as the plane takes that first dip. You are traveling with a friend who had to take medication to just get on the flight and now is shaking with fright. You want to comfort them, but you absorb their terror as you look at them, causing your face to flush with heat and your heart to race. Luckily, you catch your breath because you notice the flight attendants are calm and are still serving the snack mix. Now that you've borrowed the state of calm from people whose credibility you trust, you lend your calm to your friend. That's co-regulation.

Although we can co-regulate with a stranger whose credibility we trust, our sensitivity to others' feelings plays out most strongly in our closest relationships. This means you'll get dysregulated by the people you care the greatest about and, in turn, can unsettle those who rely on you the most. It also means *you hold the most power to lend your calming energy to your children.*

Occasionally make it look easy

Sometimes your child doesn't need to draw a lesson from your behavior, they only need to feel safe. If you have young children, they benefit from (naively) believing you can handle anything. If you have an older child, tween, or teen who is in extreme distress, they benefit from you seeming unshakable. In either case you transmit the message, "You'll be OK, because I'm OK." Essentially, you're a duck gliding effortlessly along the stream despite the current getting stronger and the winds picking up. How does that duck do it? Your child managing more than they can handle in the moment doesn't care! They just need to look at you and know the world is safe, predictable, and manageable. They need to believe you remain unfazed. Unflappable. Occasionally you may need to be like that duck, when your child can't yet handle the lessons you'd like to teach because of their developmental stage or current stressors.

But usually make it look real

If you make it look too easy, you might be a great co-regulator but miss the opportunity to help your child learn to self-regulate. And older children are highly sensitive to what you're really feeling. In other words, if you're faking it, they'll know it! So in the toughest times, be the duck gliding on the water, but more often be like the duck who is successfully navigating the current because its little feet are paddling like mad!

We help children learn self-control in the moment and self-regulation in the longer term when we help them understand how much work it takes beneath the surface to stay the course. You build your children's self-regulation skills when you show through your example all you do to "get to calm." Learn to be calm(er) and pass along what you've learned. You don't need to know all the answers or handle life with ease. Move through life's tougher moments as best as you can and be transparent with your children about what you're doing to stay afloat.

It's easier said than done

We all get occasionally dysregulated. The world offers ample opportunities to unsettle us, but because of how deeply we care about our families, you may become most dysregulated when something is happening within your family or to your child. The irony is that precisely when your skills as a co-regulator matter the most, it is hardest to remain calm. You may feel panicky yourself. How you manage that feeling will be the most impactful lesson for your child.

Humans are not good at figuring out how to calm themselves when they're most distressed. But self-regulation is the first step to being able to co-regulate. This is an intentional practice; learn the skills you need to settle yourself during your calm moments so they become second nature for when your emotions are flying.

Stress-management skills as the foundation of building resilience will be discussed in Chapter 19 and are detailed in the book *Building Resilience in Children and Teens: Giving Kids Roots and Wings*. While you can educate your child about an array of strategies to cope with their emotions, they'll learn them much better when they see them in action. So, what kind of things might your little feet be doing under the water to stay afloat? Get yourself to calm and your child will have an example to live by. The following are some brief thoughts to consider:

Anticipate problems (as best as possible). We all have had circumstances in our lives that make us react strongly—or painfully—to those situations. Knowing what pushes your buttons or has you relive awful memories will allow you to avoid what you can. It also allows you to pull from your internal resources and support systems when you anticipate an issue and prepare yourself in advance to confront it.

Create space. Sometimes we need to remove ourselves from a stressor to feel safe enough to calmly think. Time-outs never go out of style. Taking time and space to collect yourself allows you to bring your best self to any situation and model how to do so. It's OK to say, "Right now I'm upset so I shouldn't make any decisions or give any advice. For both our sakes, I'm going to calm down first. Then we'll talk." This positions you nicely to share what you did to get yourself to the point that you feel prepared to be thoughtful. Whatever worked for you in your time-out, share it to make it real. "I feel better and am ready to tackle this problem now that I have _____."

Exercise works. Working out uses up the stress hormones that activate our emergency systems. Running, or anything that involves quick movements, tells your body you've escaped (outrun) the danger.

Relax. The calm and emergency nervous systems run in parallel; one is turned on while the other is quiet. When the calm system is on, the emergency system quiets, and our thoughtful selves can operate. Deep, slow breathing turns on your calm nervous system. Yoga, meditation, and mindfulness all relax us through breathing exercises.

Prevent your thoughts from getting away from you. Being dysregulated is partly about losing control of thinking. There are strategies that help you "catch your thoughts" and drive away panic-driven and anxiety-provoking thoughts (see Chapter 21).

Express yourself. When feelings stay inside, they disrupt our ability to think clearly. If you use words to best organize your thoughts and feelings, you may find it useful to write or talk through what's on your mind. What works for you? Prayer? Expression through creative arts? Using dance or movement to release pent-up emotions? Tap into what helps center you and work through your emotions while doing what you love.

Join with others. Relationships are key. In Chapter 18, we'll talk about how human connection is the essential ingredient of resilience and thriving. Sometimes just being with another person is all it takes to gain strength and restore your calm.

Be compassionate with yourself

Forgive yourself when you get occasionally dysregulated; you deserve it. Further, it'll be good for you and your child to demonstrate this compassion. By doing so on your worst days, your child will learn that you will be more forgiving of them on their toughest days. We'll discuss this more deeply in Chapter 5. For now, consider that your child will more easily draw calm from you when they know that whatever is causing distress or self-doubt in them will never make you reject them. Forgiving yourself on your bad days drives this critical lesson home.

You'll parent more effectively when well regulated

A Lighthouse Parent scans the environment and properly assesses danger. But when operating from a place of fear, it's hard to see anything but danger. When operating on fight-or-flight mode, the word "no" becomes the reflexive response. We don't keep children safer even with unnecessarily tight restrictions because a fear-driven mind looking for imminent threats may miss the subtle signs that predict future problems are brewing. When calmer, you'll rise above your instinct to bubble wrap your child and ultimately remember that letting them explore the world under your watchful eyes is a better safety strategy. Furthermore, you'll recognize that while shouting "No!" momentarily quells your anxieties, it stifles opportunities for your child to explore, stretch, and grow. You'll also be much more receptive to the daily achievements of development that deserve your reinforcement.

Preparing to share your calm with your tween and teen

Being a source of calm for your child may pay off most critically during the teen years. The adolescent brain develops very rapidly with the emotional centers maturing even more quickly than the thinking centers. Our communication style can activate either an adolescent's emotional brain centers or their thoughtful centers. Because their emotional brain is so brilliant, once activated, it is hard for the thoughtful side of their brain to most effectively do its job. In simplest terms, when we use "cold communication," meaning we are calm, thoughtful, and respectful, the thinking parts of their brain will dominate. On the other hand, when we use "hot communication," meaning we are intensely emotional, angry, or condescending, their emotional brain dominates, making it difficult for them to think to their potential. Skilled co-regulators help adolescents access the full power of their minds. If you serve this role, you will be positioned to be a stabilizing force and key influencer in their life. Strategies to do this are covered extensively in my book *Congrats—You're Having a Teen! Strengthen Your Family and Raise a Good Person.* As the teen years approach, I recommend you dive deeply into learning more about this essential communication strategy.

Resilience in Action: We Are Stronger Together

Together we are stronger than the sum of our individual parts. When we gain emotional safety by relying on one another, we experience that key lesson of resilience. Lighthouse Parents are the source of security that enables their children to learn to navigate life's challenges. As your child successfully develops their self-regulation skills because they relied on your calming energy when they were most insecure, it will forge a special bond between you that will continue to strengthen. When you allow them to become secure in their footing as they grow, the bond you develop may allow you to strengthen and comfort each other for years to come.

CHAPTER 4

Recognize How Your Child Is Comforted

Children don't come with instruction manuals on how to comfort them in their moments of distress, but they do teach us what they need. When you observe the signals your child sends about when and how to comfort them, you'll learn how to become their source of security. How your child first settles and then calms is linked to their temperament and will change little over time. However, their developmental needs will evolve. You'll first be someone your child relies on entirely for comfort. Then, you'll help your child learn to comfort themselves, knowing they have your support as needed. Ultimately, you hope to have a mutually reliant adult relationship where you draw comfort from each other.

Your flexibility in how you comfort your child will be critical as they approach the tween years. Because your adolescent will sometimes need to push you away to see what they can handle on their own, it's important to check in on their needs rather than jump in too quickly. Some adolescents welcome your involvement immediately, while others resent parents trying to "fix" them. Most adolescents have some days they want to draw you near, and other days when they want to practice more independence. But it's always important that your involvement helps your tween or teen see themselves as a problem-solver instead of believing you see them as a problem to be solved.

Advice for parenting a child of any age: Show them with your presence that you stand by them. Then, ask them what they need from you in the moment.

Preparing for Adolescence

Adolescence is a time of intense emotions and your child may be surrounded by people who think they know the right thing to say or do to support them but miss the mark because they don't *really* know your child. You do. Your knowledge of what it takes to comfort your child will ensure they turn to you for comfort during the tween and teen years.

Shaping Your Lifelong Bond

You never get too old to draw comfort from the person who knows you best. Essential temperament characteristics don't change much over time, even if adults can better adapt to varied situations. Your adult child will likely always welcome you in their life as the person who *really* understands their needs.

Understand Your Child's Temperament

Temperament is essentially "a way of being" that influences how we deal with emotions, calm or regulate our behavior, or respond in unfamiliar situations and around new people. Some people are more emotionally reactive than others and feel their feelings with more intensity. Reactive people may be exuberant and a pleasure to be around but also find it tougher to restore themselves to a calm state. Some people find it easier to regulate their emotions and to focus on a task while others find it harder to thoughtfully consider their actions and return to their baseline after being agitated. Sociable people can enter new environments with comfort while others need to observe before dipping their toe into the water. Knowing your child's temperament prepares you to be a greater source of support because you'll better predict how they'll respond to emotional challenges or changes in their environment.

Understanding your child's temperament helps you realize much of their behavior is neither right or wrong but rather just how they are wired. You can more easily remain patient when you don't try to change something that can't—and shouldn't—be changed. Instead, you can adjust your approaches to better meet your child's needs. For example, rather than telling a reactive child to settle down when excited, we can give them needed space to work out their energy. Rather than telling a reserved child to "just introduce yourself" to make friends in a new school, we can prepare their teachers to know they slowly warm up but make a good and caring friend once comfortable. Further, when you view a misbehavior as temperament related rather than intentional, you'll react less negatively. This doesn't mean you should excuse misbehavior but rather allows you to understand its roots, which better positions you to correct it.

Knowing your own temperament can help you better understand your frustration if your child's temperament doesn't match your own. They are not trying to reject your attempts at consoling or correcting them; they may just have a different way of navigating the world and your first attempts might be based on what would work for you, not necessarily them.

How does your child react to distress?

If you can clearly describe a consistent pattern your child takes to settle, their temperament likely plays a role in how they experience and manage distress. Knowing this allows you to become a trusted source of security to them. They'll trust you because they feel understood by you. **They'll come to you most consistently when they see you know their pattern and are open to comforting them in the way that works best for them.**

Some children send their distress signals clearly, essentially screaming through their words or actions, "I need you now!" Other children keep us guessing and we need to give them space and look for subtle cues as we wait for their invitation for us to offer them support. You can't miss the children who scream for support. But we must take special care to notice distress signals from children who convey them more subtly or their needs will go unmet.

Work through the following questions to see what patterns you've noticed in your child and their temperament:

What tends to distress your child?

- Is your child most distressed in social situations, including school? Or most uncomfortable when they feel lonely?
- Does your child require consistency and predictability to feel comfortable?

- Do unfamiliar settings generate anxiety?
- Does your child get most uncomfortable if they feel they've disappointed or angered someone? Or is your child most likely to become disappointed in themselves?
- How does your child react to failure?
- Does your child experience feedback as criticism?

What does it take for your child to settle their emotions?

- Does your child distract themselves from something that upsets them by diving into a new activity?
- Does your child need space and distance to settle? If so, what signals do they send that they are ready for you to approach?
- Does your child self-soothe until they are ready to invite someone else in? If so, how have you learned to enter their world? Do you wait for an invitation or tell them you're available?
- Does your child slow down and withdraw when they are full of feelings? Or do they become active and seem to have endless energy to burn off?
- Is your child inconsolable when hungry but calmer when fed?
- Is your child more likely to fall apart if they're tired? (This is true for a lot of people!)
- Does your child have to cry it out before they talk it out?

How does your child let you know they are distressed?

- Does your child withhold any distress from you if they think you are already upset or overburdened? If so, refer to our discussion in Chapter 2.
- Is your child clear about when they need your attention, or do they leave you guessing?
- Does your child get deflated as if the energy leaves their body when they are upset?
- Does your child speak their feelings, or do you notice a change in their mood first? How do they respond to gentle questioning?
- Does your child better express what they are feeling through spoken words, writing, or creative expression, like art or song?

- Does your child become sweeter to draw you in? Or become angry, irritable, or off-putting to make sure you know they are upset?
- Does your child have physical symptoms like bellyaches or headaches even before they understand their mood has changed? (Note: Your pediatrician will consider medical concerns before concluding this is stress related. If it is stress related, this is not your child faking it or an attempt to get your attention. Rather it is related to the real connection between human emotions and our bodies.)

How does your child like to be comforted?

As we consider how your child likes to be comforted, remember that these areas may change as your child develops and trials greater independence. You also might find that your child is comforted differently depending on what has upset them. Be ready to vary your approach to the circumstance.

- Does your child come right to you and crave physical contact, like a hug, to get to calm?
- Does your child need space to process on their own? If so, make a clear statement like, "I know that you are sad. I'm here for you when you need me"?
- Does your child like you to listen to their feelings first? (Listening is an art form; see Chapter 10). Is you being present all they need?
- Does your child like to engage in an activity with you, to distract them from their feelings?
- Does your child like to speak to you through the creative arts, perhaps drawing out their feelings in a picture?
- Does your child like you to guide them through solutions? If so, do this in a way that doesn't feel like a lecture but helps them to problem-solve (see Chapter 11).

Tips to Follow and Pitfalls to Avoid

There isn't a one-size-fits-all approach that will work for comforting your child every time, but your steady presence and commitment to helping your child know they are not alone in their journey is *always* part of the solution. The following are thoughts on effective strategies to help children learn to manage their feelings. The table also includes strategies to avoid, because while well-intentioned, they may inadvertently communicate that either you don't take their distress seriously or believe they are too fragile to learn to manage their challenging thoughts and feelings.

Tips to Calm Your Child	Pitfalls to Avoid
Stay calm. Any feelings you have will spread to your child (see Chapter 3). Be patient as they reveal their thoughts, feelings, and stories to you.	To empathize, some parents feel their children's emotions so fully that children absorb their parents' feelings and escalate their own.
Know your child's comfort zone and routinely stay within it, but help your child slowly adapt to new circumstances. Their comfort zone can stretch, and their fears will ease.	Parents instinctively shield children from discomfort. Children can't stretch into new territory if they are protected and never have the opportunity to emotionally grow.
Alert your child to a situation likely to cause distress so they can activate their coping strategies. If your child does not yet possess coping strategies to a situation, you can limit exposure (if possible) while developing these strategies.	Avoid discomfort altogether.
Remain judgment free. Communicate that no feeling is ever wrong and that uncomfortable ones can be managed.	Avoid displaying disappointment in your child's intensity of emotions.
Help validate thoughts and feelings by normalizing them. You might start conversations with, "Lots of children have feelings like . . ." or "Sometimes I feel like . . ."	Avoid saying something like, "Your brother is able to _____." Or, "I'll bet your friends never get scared of _____." This can add shame to the mix of feelings your child is already experiencing.

Tips to Calm Your Child	Pitfalls to Avoid
Talk through their anxieties. Listen to their concerns and help them avoid catastrophic thinking (see Chapter 21).	Avoid simple statements like, "You worry too much." Be careful that you don't overly reassure them by indicating there is no problem at all. An anxious child can misread denial of a problem as there must be something so big to worry about that you are ignoring it altogether.
Talk about feelings and brainstorm solutions when they are calm. They'll listen more fully and tap into their own wisdom more easily.	Don't solve problems for your child in the midst of a crisis unless there is danger to be avoided.
Create private spaces and parent-child time to think things through.	Don't settle situations in public spaces or in a crowd. That could generate shame and feel disrespectful.

Help your child trust they will get through a challenge with you by their side. They should learn to problem-solve with the safety you offer, your encouragement, and occasional wisdom.	Don't be so involved that your child sees you as a problem-fixer. This will make them reliant on you when young and may leave them resenting you when older, because they may see your overinvolvement as a barrier to their independence.
Understand that people can express feelings in ways other than words. Allow play and creative expression to tell the story.	Don't say to a child "use your words" if that is not their most comfortable tool for expression.
Help other adults understand your child's temperament so they can effectively comfort them also.	Resist hiding or making excuses for your child's avoidant or acting out behaviors with child-serving professionals (like teachers). You need them to be aware of your child's discomfort, so they'll be better prepared to help.
Notice and praise small accomplishments as your child tests and stretches their comfort zone.	Your child knows you are watching. Don't wait for your child to achieve a big conquest to notice their efforts. What feels small to you might be a major leap for them.

CHAPTER 5

Your Child Is Watching: How You Judge Tells Them How Safe It Is to Come to You

Your stable presence will be most critically protective when your child is experiencing the highest levels of distress. It may be when they experience rejection from others and struggle to accept themselves. It may be when they are ashamed of a choice they've made and want to know if they can redeem themselves. It may be when they decide to share their innermost thoughts or feelings or include you as they learn who they really are. Your love in that particular moment may be the only force reminding them that they are worthy of being loved. This depends, however, on your child choosing to come to you in that moment.

Preparing for Adolescence

Adolescence is the time of identity development, where young people struggle to answer the question, "Who am I?" It can be a time of both self-doubt and increasing self-awareness. It is often a period when feedback from peers can be painful. Your tween or teen needs someone who accepts them fully and from whom they never fear rejection. Be that person now so your teen will come to you when they need you most.

Shaping Your Lifelong Bond

When you are the person who is fully accepting of your child, you will become their lifelong source of safety and self-worth. When you model that we adults deserve self-forgiveness, your adult child will be more compassionate with themselves and be forever grateful that you shared that lesson when they were a child. When you help your child know they are worthy of love and never need to fear rejection, you will remain a central support person throughout their lives. Your life will also have moments when you question your worth, and you may have the support you gave in childhood returned to you by your adult child.

Be Careful What You Judge

If you have a relationship with your child that values communication, your child will likely talk freely about most things. But they need you the most when the topic they choose to share is serious. Whether they come to you during that critical moment is linked to whether they think you'll stand by them. They must trust that including you will not harm their relationship with you. They must know that there is no chance of rejection.

None of us are without judgments, biases, or opinions. It is OK to not like a behavior. It is expected that you'll have the strongest opinions about things you worry will hurt the person you love. The question is whether your judgment is about the behavior or the person. We must address the behavior *while* fully accepting the person. And we mustn't confuse a behavior with matters of identity that define a person. A person can choose to stop smoking for example. Our children rely on us guiding them toward safety and away from dangerous or undermining behaviors. However, a human cannot change who they are at their core. The only way to address a core issue of identity—the way a person sees themselves—is to accept the person fully without imagining your opinions can or should change the person.

Eyes are always on you

Your child is not just paying attention to how you react to them. They're paying close attention to how you respond to other situations: when the neighbor annoys you, when your boss infuriates you, when your partner frustrates you, or when their sibling disappoints or disobeys you. Do you reject their behavior or them in their entirety? Are you forgiving? Do you hold a grudge? Do you give second chances? Or once you've formed an opinion, is it hard or impossible for someone to redeem themselves? If your child sees you rejecting people, they'll be less likely to come to you with something weighing heavily on their mind. They won't take the risk of losing you.

Judgment is a 2-sided coin

Because praise is a form of judgment, it can backfire when not delivered wisely. When our children do well, we want to tell them how pleased we are with their actions, behaviors, and performances. But we must avoid communicating the message, "I am proud of you when _____," or "You made me proud because _____." If this kind of praise is how you reinforce what pleases you, you can count on your child sharing their lives with you when they repeat the performance or achieve a similar outcome. But they may not come to you when they need you most because they won't want to disappoint you.

Make sure to occasionally add a line to your praise that celebrates your relationship and the fact that you care about open communication regardless of any outcome. "I am so proud of you today because _____, but I am proudest of you because you share with me what is going on in your life." Or, "I am so pleased that things are going so well; you've earned it! And I love celebrating your successes. I want you to know that I'll also be here in those moments where not everything goes as well. You're stuck with me either way." This conveys that you want your child to come to you in good times and challenging ones.

Do you forgive yourself?

Some of us are naturally forgiving of others but harder on ourselves. This may be especially true in our families. We juggle so many balls to get it right—to strike that perfect balance of performing at work while protecting our home lives. The only thing that is predictable about having too many balls in the air is that some will drop.

Listen to this: You are deserving of self-compassion when some of those balls fall to the ground. You know it. But you may feel that you don't have the time or the bandwidth to cut yourself a break because you're too focused on getting things right for others. (I know I'm not speaking to all of you, but you know if I am speaking your truth!) As deserving as you are of self-care, self-compassion, and to be forgiving of your own frailties, you might reject my message entirely if I kept the discussion about you. That's why I'm making it about your child.

If your child sees you forgiving your own imperfections, they will learn that you will accept theirs. If your child sees that you recognize your own strengths and limitations but don't focus solely on what challenges you, they'll learn that they can rise above their own challenges. If your child learns you're compassionate with yourself, they'll know they will receive compassion from you. If your child sees you forgiving yourself when you are not your very best self, they'll never fear losing you when they share their struggles.

Your child will see you as a stable force to turn to when they most need you—when they have witnessed you accepting yourself just as you are.

Part 2
Modeling and Knowing

I choose to be a Lighthouse Parent . . . from which my children can measure themselves against.

CHAPTER 6

Modeling What It (Really) Means to Be an Adult

We all know that the one job of childhood is to grow up. Seems easy enough. But grow into what? That's the big question! No wonder children and adolescents look for every clue they can gather from every source they can find: other kids, superheroes, sports stars, social media influencers, celebrities, and especially, YOU.

Lighthouse Parents recognize that our presence allows children to imagine what it means to be an adult. We're role models 24 hours a day, 7 days a week. Like it or not. You have no choice about being a role model, but you do have lots of control over the kind of model you choose to be. When you model what it means to be a caring adult, who is considerate of how our actions affect others, you allow your child to learn what a good person looks like. When you discuss how your decisions are made with attention to their implications, you paint them a vivid portrait of thoughtfulness.

It is easier for our children to imagine being real people with actual problems who are working hard nonetheless to be good than it is to imagine being perfect. In fact, perfection doesn't exist. The best role models possess an array of strengths and flaws. Knowing this, you can exhale.

Preparing for Adolescence

Preadolescent children want to be like their parents more than anything. The lessons they'll learn about what it means to be a good—albeit complex—person will remain imprinted through adolescence. This is important to remember because in their journey toward independence, many tweens or teens stop saying, "I want to be just like you when I grow up." Two lessons to emphasize: First, be a role model early when your child is proudly taking it all in. Second, adolescents never stop viewing you as a role model even if they sometimes keep that to themselves.

Shaping Your Lifelong Bond

When you behave like the 35-, 40-, or 50-year-old you hope your child might become, that method of modeling will last throughout their lives. Critically, when you model being a real human that does the very best they can—rather than pretend to be a false model of perfection—you will give your future adult child the comfort of knowing they are OK just the way they are. This will give you permission to relate to each other adult-to-adult—imperfections and all.

Being the Reflection in Your Child's Eyes

Let's begin with an exercise to work through with other adults who care about your child. Understand that the following questions reflect my values and you can replace some with items that hold more meaning to you. Please take as much time on this reflection as you can; I hope it will better shape your approach to parenting.

For all questions, imagine your child as a 35-year-old.

Who do you want them to be in relationship to others?

- Do you hope they prioritize relationships in their life or focus more on the trappings of financial success?
- Will they create the time and space for those they love?

- Will they care about the elderly in their family?
- Will they maintain relationships with their parents? Siblings?
- Will they work on building a strong community or only pay attention to those within their own homes?
- How will they treat people who are living through hardships?
- Will they make assumptions about other people or choose to learn about them directly through respectful listening?
- How will they react to people who have hurt them emotionally, treated them badly, or offended them in some way?

What character strengths do you hope they possess?

- Will they see honesty as a core value?
- Will they operate with integrity, trying to live by their ethical or moral principles?
- Will they commit to contributing to their community?
- Will they care about justice and fairness?
- Will they be open-minded and approach life with curiosity?
- Will they maintain the type of humility that leaves them open to learning from others, even those with whom they might not agree?
- Will they have a personal sense of meaning and believe they pursue a purpose?

How do you hope they attend to their well-being?

- How will they respond to stress?
- Will they turn to friends or family for emotional support?
- Will they seek professional guidance when they deserve extra support?
- Will they get adequate sleep?
- Will they take time for themselves or only give to others even at personal self-sacrifice?
- Will they know how to relax?
- Will they incorporate exercise into their routines?
- Will they appreciate nature? Animals?
- What will their relationship be with drugs and alcohol?

How would you like to see them recognizing their own strengths?

- Do they recognize themselves as worthy of being loved? As deserving of being seen in their best light?
- Will they recognize themselves as essentially a good, if imperfect, person?
- Will they comfortably acknowledge a positive attribute and help others know what skills or strengths they possess?
- Will they allow themselves to build on those strengths to optimize their contribution to a project/work environment/home/community? Or will they focus instead on their limitations and forego the unique contributions they could add?

How would you like them to respond to failure or to their own limitations?

- Will they feel as though they must always know the right thing to do?
- Will they condemn themselves every time they experience a problem?
- Will they always seek growth, or will a disappointment lead them to give up easily?
- Will they see setbacks as opportunities to do better the next time around?

How will they make decisions?

- Will they act selfishly or consider others' needs?
- Will they exhibit self-control and consider long-term implications, or will they always live for the moment?
- Will they wait to make important decisions until calm or respond impulsively when stressed?
- Will they make decisions independently or seek counsel and guidance from others who may have more experience with the matter?

Once you've considered who you want your child to be, you have the starting point to understanding who you should be as a role model. You are the model of an adult most likely to shape who they become. In other words, when we see ourselves through the reflection in our children's eyes, our vision about who we should be sharpens.

Human Role Models Are Imperfect

You know who I want to be? I want to be the person reflected in JoJo, my scruffy dog's big brown eyes. If only I was a fraction as good a person as she seems convinced I am. It's important that parents know how critical they are in shaping their children's views of what it means to be an adult. But it's also so much pressure! Some of our best opportunities to be a role model are offered when our children can see how we respond to life's most challenging moments. We discussed in Chapter 3 how our children learn to best regulate their emotions, thoughts, and feelings not when we look like we are unphased but when we demonstrate the steps we take to manage life's curveballs. We discussed in Chapter 5 how critically important our own self-compassion is to earn our children's trust that we will stand by them when they need us the most. When they see us as nonjudgmental and forgiving of ourselves in difficult situations, it helps them know we will support them in their toughest moments.

Go back to the questions listed in the previous exercise and note how many of them are about struggling to do the right thing when it isn't easy to do. They are about looking for support and doing the hard work of staying well. They are about gaining strength from relationships and contributing to others' lives. They are about committing to our own well-being, especially during stressful times.

Model self-care

Committing to self-care is a strategic act of effective parenting. When we care for ourselves we think more clearly and better regulate our emotions. We can explain this perhaps by saying, "You need me at my very best right now. I'm going to take a few moments for myself and then I'm all yours." But even without our explanation, our children will likely notice how much better we feel and how effectively we think and manage problems after we take the time for self-care.

Setting your own needs aside does not model for your child how adults sustain strength. Attending to your own well-being demonstrates that when we as humans care for ourselves, we maintain the energy to care for others as well. Critically, as discussed in Chapter 2, your children will be relieved when they know you invest in your own wellness and will come to you more freely when they don't see you as overburdened.

Lighthouses are seen

The lighthouse metaphor reminds us that we must be visible to serve our mission. Our children and teens are always watching us, but depending on their developmental level, they may or may not gain what we hope from only observing our actions. The following are a few general things you can do to make sure your children fully grasp the behaviors you hope to model.

- Children of every age, from toddlers to teens, sense their parents' state of well-being. They are more relaxed when they see you at ease and experience tension when they see you in distress.
- Over time, older children and adolescents learn to associate what kind of things affect their parents' well-being. In response, they may learn to mimic those things that seem to bring comfort to their parents and avoid those things that cause them distress.
- Older children and adolescents benefit from you processing out loud what you are experiencing. Statements like the following are ways to start conversations and to underscore your experience:
  - I feel so stressed or upset when _____.
  - To feel better when I am upset, I _____.
  - I really messed up, but I learned from it, and in the future I'll _____.
  - I really cherish helping our neighbor _____, because neighbors support each other and that builds a better community.
  - I could make it easier on myself if I just _____, but that wouldn't be living up to my values.
  - I enjoy my work, but I am always happy to come home to the people I care about.
- Young people of any age will embrace a chance to talk about or to relate a conversation to their own life. Conversations starters might include
  - You saw how that situation made me feel. How do you think you would have reacted if the same thing happened to you?

- In case I am making it look easy, let me tell you, it's not. Every time I fail, I have to remind myself I'm a work in progress who's still learning. Do you do that, or do you get down on yourself?
- Choosing to be a good person isn't always easy. Sometimes it means setting aside your own desire to feel pleasure in the moment. We all wrestle in our head. When you are working to do the right thing, what thoughts come to your mind?

Although conversations can be fruitful, the best way to help a child clarify their own values is to say little, listen, and be a sounding board. When your child takes the lead, you can ensure you are having conversations at the developmental level and pace they are prepared to handle.

Create meaningful connections

It is unrealistic—and too much pressure—to think it is only on you to model what it means to be an adult. As our children have wider exposures, they are more likely to find inspiration in other areas of their life, as well as in other people they meet. Their interests will be sparked by someone who is pursuing the same passion or helping your child pursue their passion. Further, as young people hone their values and interests, they seek others with shared thoughts and feelings who can help them imagine next steps in their development. Most people don't "apply" to be role models; they are found. Our job is to encourage our children to find those healthy role models.

Young people tend to mimic things that they consider acceptable to the community, not just to their parents. This is especially true for adolescents who are finding their identity and doing what feels "normal" to them. If they exist in a community where people hold the values you want reinforced in your child, they'll have a positive view of normal. Encourage your child to engage in activities that reflect their values, such as community or religious activities, athletics, after-school programs including sports, or volunteering in settings that reinforce the good they can do in the world.

In these settings, they'll meet both positive adult *and* peer role models. To reinforce the learning from positive (adult or peer) role models, discuss with your child what qualities they most admire in them.

Reinforce the lessons—good or bad

Role models can also negatively influence your children's view of what adulthood should look like. Some public figures, for example, might be greatly talented but make poor personal choices or reinforce hatred or division. It's not possible to shield your child entirely from negative influences. You can, however, help them process what they are seeing so they'll be able to wisely chart their own path. A simple conversation (with listening!) can include the fact that all people have both good and bad qualities, and all of us make mistakes. We are all human. Our goal is to take ownership over our mistakes, grow from them, and make amends when we have hurt others. We can also use observations of negative behaviors to underscore the point that even if we generally admire someone, we do not need to follow their lead entirely. We all choose our own behaviors. Most critically, use negative role-modeling as opportunities to allow your child to clarify what they might do differently.

CHAPTER 7

Seeing All That Is Good and Right in Your Child: The Measure They'll Use to See Themselves

Young people hear too many undermining messages about who they already are or might become. *Look this way. Act that way. Do what we do. Fit into this box. You are _____.* This chatter makes them vulnerable to influences that can lead them astray or change the way they see themselves. This unhelpful input has long been heard in schoolyards and communities, but now social media is intensifying the pressure. Your child needs you as a source of stability they can turn to as they consider who they *really* are. They gain security and protection when they see themselves as the reflection in your eyes. Knowing this, what you see matters!

Are "Good" and "Right" Judgmental Terms?

In Chapter 5, we discussed the importance of not being judgmental. The word "good" itself can at first glance feel very much like a judgmental word. "Good" can be the opposite of "bad." In fact, "right" can be interpreted as the opposite of "wrong." As a Lighthouse Parent, your strength-based approach—*really* knowing who your child is at their core—is deeply protective. These terms, therefore, are not meant as terms of judgment but, rather, as terms of *truly knowing* your child. It is about seeing the essence of who they really are. Rather than being judgmental, seeing the "good" and "right" in your child is the underpinning of genuine acceptance.

You contribute to your child's lifelong well-being when you see all that is good and right within them. The self-worth they gain will make them more likely to thrive in the best of times and prevail through the most demanding moments. They will always know that the person who knows them the most—you—sees them as good to their core and worthy of being loved. The power of that protection is incalculable. It will contribute to a deep-seated sense of security. In turn, their self-worth will allow them to give generously of themselves and value others. Their ability to do so is the foundation of meaningful friendships and healthy romantic relationships.

Preparing for Adolescence

Adolescents are natural explorers. They try on many hats to see which might best fit them. Many tweens and teens are highly sensitive to feedback from peers and can therefore choose behaviors to please them. You know them best. When you commit to seeing the best in them during childhood, they'll always be able to search for your lighthouse beam to remind themselves who they really are—and want to be.

Shaping Your Lifelong Bond

The desire to please others or do what it takes to fit in does not end with adolescence. Your adult child may best stick to their values when they are clear about who they are at their very best. No matter their age, they will retain a clear memory of how the person who knew them best—you—saw them. When you retain this positive view of your child's essence, don't be surprised when your adult child searches for that lighthouse beam as a source of reaffirmation.

Seeing Your Child as They *Really* Are

Be your child's lighthouse—someone they can look back toward when they need a reminder of who they *really* are. What do I mean by the phrase "who they really are"? Too often children and teens are judged by certain behaviors. Adults may take mental shortcuts and think that a particular behavior defines the child instead of it being a child's response to an emotion or experience. In the worst case, that child might adopt the "shortcut" themselves and see themselves as defined by the behavior. If this happens, they'll repeat the behavior often and end up acting just as people expected they might.

Some of your child's greatest strengths have always been present. Remember your pride as their core values were revealed? Maybe it was when your child chose to share, even if by giving something away it meant they would have less of it themselves. Their empathy was revealed when they nestled in your arms when you were upset. I saw this empathy in my own child years ago, when I circled back to pick up the discarded pink teddy bear on the road because my daughter knew it was sad and lonely and would feel better after a bath. Think about when signs of mental toughness, such as their commitment to stick to their beliefs, revealed themselves. You may not have liked their stubbornness, but you were able to recognize with pride that your child could stand up for themselves.

Nobody displays all their strengths at once; we all have good and not-so-good days. And many of these strengths develop over time. Your goal is to see what is good and right in your child and to support them as they grow into their best selves—not to imagine them as perfect. The following list includes strengths worth noticing. Your child likely possesses many strengths not included here, so please add to the list!

- **Honesty:** Does your child share what they truly believe? Do they do so to remain faithful to their own values? If so, they'll more likely have the kind of open communication with people where everyone's needs are understood.
- **Insight:** Does your child understand the feelings that drive their actions? Being able to grasp their behaviors, thoughts, or feelings can help them develop solutions that will work for them. They also may better understand what drives others and hopefully be more empathetic toward them.
- **Wisdom:** Is your child wise beyond their years? Do they endlessly ask questions to try to figure it all out, and as they do, can you see their understanding expanding? Do they share thoughts that surprise you?
- **Creativity:** Does your child have a wonderful imagination? Do they see things others seem not to notice? Do they express themselves in unique ways? Creative people find solutions others may overlook.

- **Secure in their differences:** Is your child someone who doesn't feel the need to fit in with what's popular? Do they know they are different and like themselves just as they are? There are so many ways humans can learn and contribute. It is a deep strength when a person can see themself as a valued and successful person, without needing to regularly compare themself to others.
- **Sensitivity:** Does your child feel richly and more fully than others? If so, they are destined to support others throughout their lives. But they also might experience pain more intensely. Helping them learn how to manage the depth of their feelings—and to see it as a strength—will be important during tough life events.
- **Compassion:** Does your child care for and about others? If so, this will bring them a sense of belonging and they may more easily find a sense of meaning and purpose. They will see painful circumstances in others' lives and choose to lend a hand. They will notice larger societal problems like poverty and homelessness and seek out the solutions we need.
- **Respect:** Does your child listen in a way that people feel heard? Do they respect earned wisdom and understand that each person deserves to be valued? People who approach personal or professional relationships in a respectful manner will have more productive conversations and form more meaningful connections.
- **Fairness:** Has your child been the kind of person who always had a sense that not everyone was treated fairly? Were they more patient waiting in line than most children because they knew others deserve a turn too? When they are rewarded with something special, do they look at those who didn't and decide to share? People with a genuine sense of fairness can better resolve conflicts and will be sought after to manage problems now and in the future.
- **Humor:** Does your child's humor enable them to get through the bumps and bruises of life? A sense of humor can often keep things in perspective. And others will enjoy being around them even in challenging moments.
- **Wonder:** Does your child possess a sense of awe that allows them to appreciate life's simple and great pleasures? If so, they'll never stop learning, and that will contribute to lasting joy and appreciation.
- **Gratitude:** Does your child appreciate what they are given? Grateful people also may be more generous with others because they know they have much to share.

- **Loyalty:** Does your child stand up for people they care about and protect others who need their support? People who learn the benefit of supporting others are often rewarded with loyalty in return.
- **Protectiveness:** Does your child sense danger and steer others away from it? Did a difficult life help them earn this protective nature? We certainly don't want our children to experience hardship, but this well-earned protective nature will benefit the relationships in their lives.
- **Perseverance and drive:** Does your child seem to never give up? If someone suggests they can't do something, do they double down to prove that they can? Children who learn to maintain a sharp focus on what they hope to achieve are more likely to reach their goals.
- **Resourcefulness:** Does your child make the effort to find what they need? Can they stretch their resources or wisely engage others to meet their needs? Resourceful people can better thrive in scarce times, often by pooling their resources with others.
- **Resilience:** Does your child grow from rather than being defeated by life's curveballs? Have they been through tough times but instead of harboring anger remain exceptionally loving? Children who learn to recover from hard times can use these coping skill sets when similar situations arise.

You'll be amazed by the strengths your child has always possessed. Be sure to show how proud of them you are in how their strengths grow as they continue to find and develop new ones.

Telling your child you like what you see

Recognizing your child's strengths does more than help them have healthy self-esteem. It elevates and reinforces all that you appreciate about them. Too often, praise highlights superficial characteristics, such as appearance or performance. In this chapter, we focus on something much more meaningful than praise. We focus on recognizing core strengths and values in your child. Often, you'll notice their strengths as they draw from them. Point them out when you see them in action.

"Your compassion is what drove you to stand up for that boy in your class who was being teased."

Even a reaffirming nod or glint in your eye will tell your child that you see and celebrate that value within them.

Your child must know you love what you see, even when you don't always see them behaving their best. Loving them unconditionally while acknowledging both their strengths and challenges offers the truest security. This becomes the root of their resilience. Loving fully doesn't mean you have to like everything they do. You can dislike their behavior at times. In fact, you can reject a behavior precisely because you fully embrace them as a human and understand the behavior does not reflect them as a whole.

Always leave room for error

Seeing your child positively is protective, unless it feels like pressure to them. Focusing on strengths can backfire when we expect our children to always behave in a positive manner. Humans can't be expected to be flawless. As you focus on their strengths, be certain that it doesn't feel as though there is a condition placed on your acceptance. Children who believe they're only accepted when they are "good" may develop anxiety or a fear of failure. See the first section of the following chart for some affirming statements and others worth avoiding. Notice that some of the statements in the second column of the chart seem affirming but actually place a condition on acceptance.

Say This	Not That	Because
You make me proud when _____.	You disappoint me when you don't _____.	Reinforcing the positive is a productive strategy that avoids instilling guilt.
I noticed that you were _____.	Why don't you ever _____?	Many children don't know we notice their positive behaviors and find it reaffirming when we do. The second statement suggests we are comparing them to others and left disappointed.
You make a difference when _____.	If only you would _____.	Noticing the effects of a positive action reinforces it. The second statement expresses disappointment.

It's Nice to Say	Try Not to Say	Because
I love it when _____. Nobody's perfect and I'll still love you when you're not always able to _____. But I sure do appreciate the effort you're putting in.	You please me because you always _____.	Children deserve reinforcement of positive behaviors but also need to know that we don't "always" expect them. Otherwise, they may develop a fear of rejection when they are not at their best.
I see you. And I like what I see!	When you do _____, I really like it.	The word "when" places a condition on your acceptance. This can lead to a child or teen fearing coming to you when they are not doing what you like. Critically, this may be when they need you the most (See Chapter 8, the part titled "Having Your Child's Back").
You're not having the best day. We all have those days. You'll do better tomorrow!	I know you can do better! Your behavior today is disappointing.	We want our children to know we all have bad days. The problem with the phrasing in the second column is that children may not hear the word "today" and may hear that their behavior is consistently disappointing.

Don't only notice strengths when your child is behaving well. Our deepest strengths are often revealed in challenging moments. These strengths may not *yet* have matured enough to be experienced in the way we'd hope. For example, sensitive children may be hurt more deeply or react more strongly to something another child could easily move past. You might see brooding, or even rage, but underneath those emotions is a hurting human. You are positioned to be supportive when you notice their sensitivity rather than view them as ill behaved. This may especially pay off during adolescence when emotions can be heightened. You want your child knowing how to manage those emotions instead of taking steps to dampen them (eg, through substance use). This concept is covered in-depth in my book *Congrats—You're Having a Teen! Strengthen Your Family and Raise a Good Person.*

Steering Away From Problems by Building on Strengths

Seeing your child in the best light is key to their positive development but is also the strongest tool in your toolbox to prevent them from being derailed. When you dislike a behavior, reinforce that you know who your child really is. Simply say, *"I know you can _____, because you have always _____."* For example, *"I know you can be gentler with your sister. I've seen how protective you can be of her, like when she is being teased by others. She needs that kindness now."* In challenging times, your knowledge of your child's strengths will ground them in who they want to be. They'll remember how right it feels for them when they make you proud by being themselves.

It is the accountability we hold for our children to be their best selves that buffers them against negative or undermining forces. Our high expectations are a critical counter force to peer pressure and discriminatory messages. Our unwavering high regard gives them the drive to push forward against low expectations. If our children are seen through the lens of a mistake they have made or a behavior that doesn't reflect who they *really* are, knowledge of their worthiness and potential reminds them of their better selves. Most vitally, it reminds them of the standards to which they should hold themselves.

Focusing on strengths may count most when times are tough

Being a Lighthouse Parent means that you offer a safe and stable place to return. It is unrealistic to believe that any close and meaningful relationship will be without challenges or to assume the journey to adulthood can entirely avoid some bumps and bruises. In Chapters 32 and 33, we consider how our knowledge of our children's essential strengths will support their resilience in trying times, help to restore our relationships after family conflict, and bring them back to safe behaviors after they have strayed into dangerous territory.

Part 3

Communicating

I choose to be a Lighthouse Parent . . . I'll send my signals in a way they will choose to trust.

CHAPTER 8

Your Unwavering Presence Offers Powerful Protection

A lighthouse is present. Stable. Constant. Predictable. No matter how thick the fog or turbulent the waters, when one sees the light in the distance, one calms and regains a sense of security. *The lighthouse communicates its power and protection through its presence.*

This may be the most important chapter in this book. Don't let its length confuse you; they're not a lot of tips and tricks needed to just show up. It's about listening well (see Chapter 10). Generally, it's about what you communicate without words, and occasionally through carefully chosen words (see Chapter 11).

Preparing for Adolescence

Children feel secure when they know their parents will remain present and stick by them no matter what. We reinforce this when we show up without ready-made answers and allow our children to guide us in how we can best support them. This will pay off in adolescence when your child may navigate many pushes and pulls but ultimately turn to you for guidance knowing you'll always stand by them.

Shaping Your Lifelong Bond

Your adult child will not remember everything you said or did during their childhood, but they will remember whether they felt more secure in your presence. They'll remember whether they could consistently rely on you or only come to you when they were certain they would please you. Parenting with unwavering presence and unconditional support may be the surest way of ensuring your adult child will often desire your presence.

But What Do I Say?

Over the decades, countless parents have asked me to supply them with the "right" words they can use to resolve a problem their child is experiencing. My answer is consistent: *Show up and stand by your child. Then, listen to learn what your child needs.* Do they just need you to be a sounding board? Do they need a reminder that you're not going anywhere—that you would never reject them? Does your presence reinforce that the person who knows them best—all their strengths, challenges, and complexities—chooses to love them? What could possibly be more protective than that?

Show up and then ask for direction

Once you've shown up, what should you do then? *Ask.* It's as simple as that. Ask whether your child wants an embrace. Ask if they just want your quiet but undeniable presence or an ear to work through their feelings. Ask if they want guidance or space *for a moment.* That moment may seem like forever when you want to move into rescue mode, but with that pause you're ultimately conveying trust. You trust that they'll get through this by drawing from their strengths—their ability to comfort themselves and ultimately find solutions—with you standing steadfast and ready by their side. Knowing that you are an "ask" away is enough to assure they will find the strength to get through their struggles.

I have been privileged to partner with SpeakUp!, a remarkable organization in the Philadelphia region that brings youth, educators, and parents together for open, honest conversations that lead to stronger relationships (https://speakup .org). Part of SpeakUp!'s power is that it gives youth the opportunity to offer adults direction about how to best support them. Underscoring the importance of parents being present and just listening, these youths shared the following:

"We want to be heard before we are helped."

"When you trust us, we trust ourselves."

"Just ask us, 'Do you want advice, or do you just want to vent?'"

"What helps is when parents listen and educate themselves more than trying to fix (our problems). When we open up about issues, our parents tend to offer advice we don't want. I only want them to hear me out and comfort me. I know it is hard because they are used to being the problem-solver."

"We expect our parents to be perfect, but this is their first time raising you. They don't always know what to do. They want to help but don't know how you want to be comforted so it comes down to communication. Parents, just ask your child how you can be helpful. Ask what they want and need."

Having your child's back

When I speak to young people about what they really need from someone, especially their parents, they say they need to know someone *really* has their back. What does that mean? They say it's clear that when things are going well they have a cheering section behind them, but it's not as clear when things are not going well that they will still be supported.

Adults are often terrific cheerleaders. When our children report a wonderful accomplishment, like doing well in school, we congratulate them on their achievement. We also praise them when they've behaved in a way that makes us particularly proud. Receiving cheers feels good in the moment because it's nice to be recognized for what they've earned. Scores. Grades. It also feels nice to be recognized for good behavior. Remembering how good it feels, they return for more affirmation when they repeat their successes. And the time after that. And after that.

But what happens when things don't go so well? What they initially heard was, "I'm so proud of you because of _____." When things are not going as well, they're going to remember how proud you were of them *because* of a way they behaved or something they accomplished. Out of fear of disappointing you, they may not tell you what's going on in their life precisely when they need you the most.

To really have your child's back, let them know that what gives you the greatest joy is to be closely connected to them and have a trusting relationship with them. You want to know that when things are going well, they will share it, and that when they need you the most, they'll *also* share it. Notice their accomplishments and reinforce their positive behaviors but always remember to *also* celebrate your relationship, your connection, and the fact that they trust you with the details of their lives. This will tell your children that you stand by them today in good times and that you'll stand by them tomorrow when life is challenging.

Silence is not a void

Chapters 10 and 11 are about the power of listening and about using your words wisely. One of the best ways of listening is to be *truly silent*. Your child will feel supported as long as your presence is unconditional and your love is unwavering. The right words will come when needed. Don't force them. Saying little while standing steadfast by your child can be a way of lending them your strength and of sharing your calm. Your silent presence says that things will be OK. When your child invites your active guidance, your words can then fill that space.

Say This	Not That
I'm here, I'm listening.	Tell me everything.
Do you want some space or time alone? Do you want me to just be here with you? Or would a hug help now?	Let me give you a hug.
I'm so proud of who you really are.	I'm so proud of you because you accomplished _____.
I'm so happy you came to me. (Think of many different ways to say it is the *relationship and trust* you value most.)	I'm so proud of you because you accomplished _____.
I'm so glad you've come to me when things didn't turn out the way you would have liked.	I'm so disappointed in you because you did _____.
I'm so glad you've come to me when you've found yourself in trouble.	I'm so angry with you because you did _____.
Nothing.	Answers your child is not ready for.
Nothing.	Questions your child is not ready to answer.
Nothing.	Words only to fill the space.

Long-lasting effects of showing up

Ultimately, people want to grow to make relatively independent decisions, but they never tire of human support and being cared about. If you supply answers, your children may grow to turn away from you as they learn to find their own. If your power is your presence—a presence that trusts your child as the expert in their own life—your adult child will continue to seek the comfort and stability of having a Lighthouse Parent.

CHAPTER 9

Parenting for Optimal Influence: Balance the Expression of Your Love With Setting Protective Rules

Lighthouse Parenting is rooted in the extensive research and experience that has proven balanced (aka authoritative) parenting works. I wrote this book so you have the skills to *apply* the principles we have known for decades to create the best educational, behavioral, and emotional outcomes for children and adolescents. This approach to parenting *also* strengthens families, creating the closest and most communicative relationships. I believe these points are interrelated; strong families are more likely to have children with better behavioral and emotional outcomes.

Before I move on, it must be stated clearly that even the strongest families can't prevent their children from experiencing all problems. Your strength shows when you stand by your child and teen when problems arise. The depth of your caring and commitment to support your child makes the difference in how they will fare during challenging times.

Preparing for Adolescence

Striking the right balance between expressed love and rules makes the difference between whether your child will feel cared about or controlled. Adolescents cherish loving guidance but are wired to gain independence and reject anything that feels like control.

Shaping Your Lifelong Bond

Adults should be confident in their ability to stand on their own but value interdependence and mutual reliance. Adults rightfully avoid relationships that feel controlling. When our children understand that our rules come from a place of loving guidance and not a desire to be controlling, they will more likely grow into adults who continue to seek our guidance.

Lighthouse Parenting Is Balanced Parenting

It seems that every year there are a few new approaches to parenting named after various animals, farm implements, or recreational vehicles. While new approaches to parenting grab media attention and earn online clicks, they may be confusing to parents trying to effectively guide their children. Driving the confusion is that some strategies they espouse make sense, leading reasonable parents to believe that the whole model must be effective. With few exceptions, however, those strategies don't present the full picture of what works in parenting. Developmental science and long-term experience tell us what works: **balance.**

Lighthouse Parenting guides us on how to balance our expressed love with clear expectations and firm guidelines that protect our children. Parents who achieve this balance encourage open communication and, therefore, strengthen their families. Lighthouse Parenting metaphorically presents the key elements of balanced parenting. This book is designed to tell you how to put each key element into action.

I choose to be a Lighthouse Parent. A stable force on the shoreline from which my child can measure themselves against. I'll send my signals in a way they'll choose to trust. I'll look down at the rocks to be sure they don't crash against them. I'll look into the waves and trust they'll learn to ride them, but I'm committed to prepare them to do so. I'll remain a source of light they can seek whenever they need a safe and secure return.

Balanced parenting makes a BIG difference

Parents who follow balanced parenting strategies raise children who achieve greater academic success, engage in fewer behavioral risks, possess a higher level of emotional well-being, and have reduced emotional distress. Balanced parenting leads to child outcomes related to

- Better emotional and mental health, including reduced depression and anxiety
- Higher levels of resilience
- Better self-esteem
- Improved grades and better engagement with teachers
- Increased participation in after-school and extracurricular activities
- Less experience being bullied or bullying others
- Less exposure to violence

Those benefits extend into the teen years when it has been shown to also reduce behavioral risks, including

- Less substance use
- Later start of sexual activity and safer sexual behaviors
- Safer driving behaviors and fewer car crashes

Most importantly, balanced parenting leads to the closest, warmest, and most communicative relationship in families. Balanced (Lighthouse) Parents also know more about what is going on in their children's lives and therefore can monitor them more closely (read on!).

What Is Meant by "Parenting Style"?

Parenting style describes the interplay between love (expressed as warmth), responsiveness (flexibility to adjust to changing needs), and demandingness (expectations and how rules are set and monitored). *Parenting style* was first described in the 1960s by Diana Baumrind, PhD, a distinguished developmental psychologist. Generations of psychologists since have studied its effect on raising children and teens and have generated likely the largest body of parenting research.

The 4 parenting styles

Which of the following sounds most like you?

- "You'll do what I say. Why? Because I said so!"
- "I really enjoy you. I couldn't always speak to my parents. I hope that if you think of me as a friend, you'll feel comfortable coming to me. I'll spend time with you and we'll have good times. I trust you to make your own decisions."
- "Kids will be kids. I turned out OK and so will they. I'll get involved if they get into serious trouble."
- "I love you. I'm not your friend, I am your parent, and that's even better. I'm going to let you make mistakes, but if something might affect your safety, I'll step in. My job is to keep you safe and stand by you as you grow into your best self."

You'll do what I say. Why? Because I said so! This is called *authoritarian parenting*. It focuses on rules but not on expressions of warmth. Parents who utilize this parenting approach don't want to be questioned. Its strength is that children know their parents are paying attention to them and watching their behaviors.

I really enjoy you. I couldn't always speak to my parents. I hope that if you think of me as a friend, you'll feel comfortable coming to me. I'll spend time with you and we'll have good times. I trust you to make your own decisions. This is called *permissive parenting*. It is rooted in warmth and expressions of love, but few rules are given. Permissive-style parents worry that close monitoring or enforcing limits may harm their relationships because their children will feel mistrusted. They also tend to be conflict avoidant, so they give their children a lot of room to make their own decisions. The strength of this approach is that family members tend to have warm relationships.

Kids will be kids. I turned out OK and so will they. I'll get involved if they get into serious trouble. This is called *disengaged parenting*. Disengaged parents rarely express their feelings to their children and don't watch closely over them. They may have other stressors in their life and therefore get involved only in crisis situations where they emphatically tell their children what they must do. A disengaged parent may think, "It doesn't matter what I think, they have their own minds." (It is crucial that all parents understand how much they do matter!) The strength of this approach is that it fosters independence and allows children to learn life lessons. (But . . . children consistently learn life lessons better with adult reflection and guidance.)

I love you. I'm not your friend, I am your parent, and that's even better. I'm going to let you make mistakes, but if something might affect your safety, I'll step in. My job is to keep you safe and stand by you as you grow into your best self. This is called *balanced parenting* (or *Lighthouse Parenting!*). It is high in expressed warmth and is responsive to children's individual and developmental needs. It includes clear limitations and monitoring of rules to protect children but also guides them so they are prepared to expand their boundaries. Among its many strengths are that lighthouse families have the closest relationships and openly communicate.

Why other parenting styles are less effective than Lighthouse Parenting

Children raised by *authoritarian* parents tend to be well behaved, *until* they can get past the rules. Some delay worrisome behaviors but then may participate in negative behaviors in the mid to later teen years to assert their independence. Some children raised by authoritarian parents may feel powerless to make their own choices and, in the worst scenario, seek relationships with controlling people later in life because they may have grown used to being controlled.

Children raised by permissive parents know they are loved but crave boundaries. They worry about disappointing their parents when they make mistakes. Statistics reveal they often participate in risky behaviors, perhaps because they assume they have permission to do so. Most concerning is that repeated studies reveal teens don't involve permissive parents in serious discussions. This is particularly disappointing and confusing to these parents because of how much they value close, communicative relationships. This may be because permissive parents often position themselves as "friends" with their child. The child may withhold information in order to not lose or let down their "friend." Remember that many children have experienced rejection from their friends and thus fear being judged by them. As a parent, the unwavering presence you offer is more powerful than that of friendship.

Children raised by disengaged parents often have the least desired outcomes. They may not be aware of their parents' stressors and may interpret their distance as a choice to remain uninvolved. These young people have the highest rates of misbehavior, perhaps to get their parent's attention since they've learned that their parents are most likely to dive in during crises.

Key points: Our love holds the most power when our children know how deeply we care about them. The limits we put into place are most closely followed when children know we monitor them and set rules not to control them but to keep them safe. They most comfortably follow rules when they know we want them to stretch into new territory when prepared to do so.

> "I can't allow you to _____. I need to keep you safe and to raise you to be a good person. I love you and that is why I insist on _____. I believe you can handle _____ now, and when you demonstrate that you can handle _____ later, I'll support you to take on as much as you can wisely and safely."

Responsiveness: a POWERFUL tool

One reason a balanced parenting style strengthens families is that children need and appreciate parents who are responsive to their needs. Being responsive means being flexible instead of rigid. Responsive parents recognize children's unique needs and reward their growing displays of responsibility with more independence. In contrast, parents with rigid rules may never change those rules in response to evolving circumstances or displays of increased responsibility. Their children may feel as if their efforts go unnoticed and experience rules as controlling. Responsive parenting leads to more open communication because children share their lives more fully with their parents when they know their progress and evolving maturity will be noticed and rewarded with increased privileges and responsibilities. We can make it clear we are being responsive when we notice progress and directly link it to a reward. "I notice that you have done so well with _____ and think you are ready to have even more responsibility. Do you think you can handle _____ now?"

Responsiveness is about paying attention to what your children can handle. Therefore, it is not just about increasing privileges; parents may need to place a hold on increasing responsibilities until the child has demonstrated they are thriving with their current level of responsibilities. In some cases, parents may even need to pull back on privileges because a child is not able to manage them. To make it easier to be responsive, avoid linking privileges with an age or timeline. Don't, for example, make a rule such as, "Until you are X years old," or link a privilege to "After you've done _____ for 3 months." It is wiser to link loosening or tightening of the reins to demonstrated behaviors. You might say, for example, "My goal is for you to be able to _____, and when you demonstrate that you are able to _____ successfully, we'll both know that you are ready." More on this approach in Chapter 16 when we discuss discipline. Sneak preview: "Discipline" means to teach or to guide, not to punish or control.

Preparing Your Child to Navigate Their World

The best parenting decisions are made when you account for the reality your child needs to navigate. If your child tends to push limits and take chances, your boundaries need to be firmer and your monitoring needs to be stricter. Believe it or not, young people appreciate it when we hold them accountable for undesired behavior. It reminds them that we know their potential and have high expectations for them.

If your child is exposed to undermining forces such as racism or overt hatred, your guidance *should* be given with urgency. Your clear boundaries and explicitly clear warnings may be the surest way to help them stay safe within a world that is not. Being firm or speaking with urgency does not make you an authoritarian parent if your child knows the boundaries are set because you care. If your child knows your watchfulness and restrictions are rooted in caring and a commitment to protect them, rather than a desire to restrict or control them, you are a Lighthouse Parent.

Build New Parenting Strengths

We are all trying our darndest to get this parenting thing right. Especially people who seek out parenting books! A starting place for growth in your parenting repertoire is to recognize all you are already doing right. If you recognize the positives of your current approach, you'll breathe easier because you are part-way there. And you'll more effectively partner with other adult caregivers by acknowledging their best intentions and existing strengths.

Consider how you adopted your current parenting approach, and reflect on what's been working well and what hasn't. People tend to parent like they were parented—or are adamant about doing things differently. Resolve to practice those facets of your parents' style that worked for you and adjust those that didn't. "Worked" doesn't just mean you turned out OK; it means it allowed you to grow while feeling confident in your abilities and secure in your attachment to your parents.

Let's consider your parenting strengths.

- If you currently lean authoritarian, you have a commitment to being involved in your child's life and to ensuring appropriate behavior.
- If you currently lean permissive, you care about having a warm, close, and trusting relationship with your child.
- If you are more disengaged, you respect that children learn from life lessons and gain confidence through picking themselves up.

No matter your parenting approach, embrace your cultural strengths, your community values, and the resources available to your children. Using these strengths, you can build new communication skills and parenting strategies that will help you reach that balance of warmth, watchfulness, and responsiveness.

Adding balance to an authoritarian style

You'll better meet your parenting goals if your child knows your actions are rooted in your love for them and your commitment to their safety. Continue watching closely but do so while openly sharing how much you care, and connect your caring to why you're fiercely protective. Let them know you are holding them accountable because you expect them to be the good person you know them to be. Remember, Lighthouse Parents have the most authority over their children's behaviors because their guidance and protection is welcomed.

Adding balance to a permissive style

Stay loving and communicative but make your child's life easier and more predictable by setting, explaining, and monitoring appropriate limits. If you struggle with this, remember that clear boundaries offer *more*, not less, freedom because children can safely experiment within the limits we've set. Further, remember that a "no" motivated by the desire to protect your child is an act of caring.

Adding balance to a disengaged style

Engaged parents don't diminish the power of life lessons, they underscore and solidify them. They hear their children's thoughts and experiences and then discuss feelings and consequences with them. Balanced parents don't want their children to avoid all failures, they want them to gain lessons from them, including learning how to bounce back and recover. Further, when Lighthouse Parents know their children are ready for additional life lessons, they encourage them to stretch into new territory.

Bring other adults on board

You may be sharing parenting responsibilities with another adult with a *very* different take on effective parenting. Manage your frustrations by understanding that their intentions are to do what they believe works best for your child. From there, nudge them toward a balanced approach by first recognizing the strengths of their current parenting approach. Then, ask them to consider how they could balance out their current approach. Perhaps they need to add setting limits to their permissive style, with an understanding that it is a loving act. If they lean authoritarian, perhaps they need only explain that they set rules because they are committed to protect who they love. If it helps, invite them to read this chapter to learn the proven benefits of balanced parenting.

Lighthouse Parenting Leads to More Answers

Be the kind of parent whose child *chooses* to talk to them. Asking a lot of questions doesn't always lead to truthful answers. Microchipping is immoral. Tracking your child signals distrust, and any savvy 10-year-old can get around most technology anyway. *It's not about what you ask that allows you to protect your child, it is what you know.* Lighthouse Parents practice the kind of open communication that makes their children include them in their lives. Your child or tween wants your guidance and supervision to keep them safe. But as they enter adolescence, they also want independence and do not want to feel controlled. They want you to support their need to explore but to set some boundaries when needed.

So now imagine yourself as a child. Who would you choose to help you evaluate a situation for safety? Remember, as a child, you want to safely stretch as far as you can, reject intrusion, and appreciate being cared about. You wouldn't turn to an authoritarian parent for advice or permission because you know their answer—it's "Don't!" You wouldn't turn to the permissive parent who will reflexively say, "I trust you, yes!" You wouldn't go to the disengaged parent because you have learned (perhaps mistakenly) to believe they'll just tell you, "I don't care." You would go to the Lighthouse Parent for caring advice that is mindful of both safety and your need to ultimately be prepared to explore on your own.

Words Matter

- Use your words!
- Love counts most when our children know they are loved. Don't assume they know how much you care about them.
- The boundaries we set are more closely followed when we discuss why we have them.
- Sharing how you make decisions, particularly when they're related to safety, helps your child develop their own decision-making skills.
- Hold healthy give-and-take conversations. Knowing you are *really* listening and willing to be responsive helps children develop well-thought-out safety plans to earn your trust. They are also more likely to follow rules when they know their privileges expand with demonstrated responsibility.

Resource

The Center for Parent and Teen Communication is committed to strengthening family relationships and building youth with the character strengths that will prepare them for healthy, successful, and meaningful lives. It is rooted in Lighthouse Parenting.

https://parentandteen.com

CHAPTER 10

Listen Well: It's Key to Protect and Prepare Your Child

I t's hard to listen when we have so much to say! We know our children need protecting so it seems logical to share our experiences with them, hoping they'll never repeat our mistakes. We know they aren't ready to make some of their own decisions, so telling them what to do seems like an easy shortcut. But shortcuts don't work in parenting. Developing our children's wisdom does. The best way to protect our children is to prepare them to think for themselves. But in what areas do they need support? It is also our indispensable role to serve as guides but toward what direction? It is because of these unknowns that you need to create the space for the answers to reveal themselves.

Healthy adults seek relationships with those who respectfully try to understand their thoughts and feelings. Listening sets the stage now for the kind of close adult-to-adult relationship you want with your child for decades to come. When we lead with commands or even share our opinions before being invited to do so, our presence can be resented and may be pushed away.

Preparing for Adolescence

Adolescence is a time when our children's ability to think things through is expanding at an astounding rate. For them to build these new thinking muscles they have to try out their thoughts and feelings and work through their plans. Develop the kind of relationship in childhood where your child feels heard and they'll come to you as a sounding board in the tween and teen years.

Shaping Your Lifelong Bond

No person of any age likes to be told what to do or how they should think. People like to be genuinely heard. Listen well during their childhood and you'll likely be lending an ear for decades to come. Even more so, you'll raise someone who enjoys listening to you as well.

Listening to Learn

Until recently, parents were advised to ask their child lots of questions: "Who are you going to be with? Where are you going? What will you be doing? When will you be home? Will adults be there?" It was assumed the who, what, where, when, and why questions best positioned parents to be active guides. But this strategy commonly breaks down in the teen years when adolescents can skirt the truth if they feel the questions are too intrusive. Don't use a communication strategy now that will fail in a few years. It's not what you ask, it's what you know. Teens share more with parents who listen to them than they do with ones who micromanage their lives or demand information. Help your child get in the habit of telling you their story, because they want to, and because they've learned how good it feels when someone who cares about them listens attentively and guides them wisely.

Sometimes, talk quickly!

When your child was a preschooler, you didn't allow them to touch the stove, nor did you let them run into traffic. If it's a "hand on the stove" moment, there isn't time to talk, and an immediate reaction is necessary. Sometimes it's hard to discern a "hand on the stove" moment from one that terrorizes us. It's hard to watch children make mistakes because we want to prevent the distress we know may follow. Breathe. If it's physically dangerous or emotionally irreparable, jump in. Otherwise, know that lessons learned are deeply imprinted and your wisdom has more staying power when you guide your child on how to make wiser, safer decisions.

Strong reactions (of any kind) shut down communication

The hard work of listening begins by avoiding communication traps that give your feelings away too easily. Children may stop talking when parents fill in the space with words or react too quickly. The first trap to avoid is the "parent alarm," driven by fear that your child is in danger. You may jump to the rescue before you've understood the issue. "Mom, Liam is being mean to me," may trigger you to respond with, "He's a bully, I'm calling his parents." This reaction would miss the opportunity to hear why your child's feelings were hurt in their own words. It may not be bullying at all but an opportunity to learn what your child is sensitive about. If there is bullying, the story will still unfold if you withhold your initial reaction. When your internal parent alarm blares, instead of going into rescue or fix-it mode, allow your child to problem-solve with your guidance.

Alarm signals can be triggered when our own experiences generate fear that our child may relive pain we've experienced. Hardships you've endured may have earned you the right to assume the worst, but it won't help you parent. Ask yourself, "Am I reliving my own experience? Do I really know what is going on here?" Then remind yourself that you can be most helpful if you learn what is going on first. This might be enough to quiet your racing mind and give you the strength to pause and listen.

Strong displays of empathy can also shut down communication. If your child believes they are causing you sadness or pain, they'll stop sharing out of fear of hurting you. This may be especially true if you've had a difficult or challenging life, and your child (no matter the age, trust me) feels a need to protect you. Sometimes we express empathy by jumping in to take our child's side. You might agree their teacher is unfair or their friend doesn't deserve them. The problem here is that their feelings may be fleeting and they may just need a moment to vent. But when you jump in too quickly, you lock them into a position they might have trouble retreating from or may be too embarrassed to tell you they know they messed up. Critically, as we discussed in Chapter 5, they may hold back in the future from coming to you when they need you the most out of fear of being rejected, just as they see you quickly taking sides against—or rejecting—someone who has hurt them. Ask, "What will be most helpful here? Do you just need to share what happened, or do you want me to think this through with you?"

Praise feels nice but can be a communication trap because it's still judgment even if the judgment is good. A sensitive young person could create an internal message after being praised: "This is what I *must* do to please my parent, and if I don't, I'll disappoint, be judged, or feel rejected by them." Use praise to share how pleased you are that they're talking more than focusing on the specific content they're saying. Also, praise the effort it took them to accomplish something. Say something like, "You worked hard and I'm proud." Avoid, "You make me proud when _____," because the underlying message might feel like, "You might not make me proud if you don't _____."

Be a sounding board

Parents often struggle to find the right words when their children are in distress. They worry their advice will not fit or their words will offer little comfort. Don't worry about providing solutions. Be there. Show up. Be a sounding board and help them work through it. When you choose to be a sounding board, you reinforce that your child is the expert in their own life and that the solutions reside within them. This is true even for a young child and especially true for a teen. What changes is the depth of their insight and the level of guidance they require. People of any age (even you!) who are stressed operate on survival mode driven by emotions, rather than on problem-solving mode. When we serve as a sounding board, we create the safe space and comfort that allows children to destress. Operating from a calmer place, they can access their internal wisdom at a pace that suits them and invite us to offer them the lessons life has given us.

You are a sounding board when you create a space free from interruptions or reactive judgment. You offer guidance when asked and allow your child's ideas to bounce around in your presence. This space allows their thoughts to become organized and to consider how their plans could play out. Not reacting is the hardest thing you might do as a parent. But the stability you offer with your nonjudgmental presence is precisely what offers the security for them to access their own wisdom and comfortably express their thoughts and feelings.

We usually think of a sounding board as something that allows words to bounce off. But many children may not express themselves best through words. Your child may be more of an artist or a performer, revealing their thoughts and feelings through nonverbal expression. Listen with the same level of intensity and passion as you would with well-formed words or expression of tears. Avoid the communication trap of telling them precisely how you interpret their artistic expression. Ask clarifying questions like, "When you show me _____ (ie, art, music, dance, or another creation) it makes me feel deeply. What does it do for you?" Even with this prompting, your child may not be able to express their thoughts through words. Be satisfied if they learn that their expression engaged you. Knowing you appreciated them sharing will hopefully motivate them to continue revealing themselves.

But wait, doesn't a good parent judge?

A parent should always be assessing for safety and determining how they should guide their child. They should also have values they hope their child will care about and behaviors they desire their children follow. The focus on being nonjudgmental does not suggest you shouldn't convey high standards. When your child was 3 and saw the world as good or bad, it was precisely your clear instructions that molded them. Your older child should also know your rules about behavior.

It is of unparalleled importance, however, that your child never fears losing you because you've judged something they've done, thought, or felt. It must be clear to them that you will always accept your child. Withholding judgment is a communication strategy that allows you to hear the full story. Once you reveal judgment, your child may stop sharing their experiences and often shut down. After you've heard their story and are grounded in an understanding of what is going on, then ask permission to share your thoughts. If you've listened fully, your child will be ready to access your wisdom and experience.

When we listen, we create a safe space for the person being heard. This is always nice, but is critically important when the other person may be feeling insecure or experiencing emotional pain. If your relationship is to endure for decades, your child should learn that your guidance is helpful in navigating their struggle and that you being a safe person in their life—one who will never reject them—is unquestioned.

Words that convey "I'm listening"

Let go of the habit of listening for pauses in conversation so you can add your own opinion. Your actions demonstrate your commitment to listening. Sit quietly, turn off your phone, and set aside distracting tasks. But there are also key words that demonstrate listening matters to you. Some phrases may feel strange at first; practice can make them feel and sound more conversational. First, remember the absence of words—silence—sends the clear message that you value that your child is speaking. It doesn't mean you agree with everything said but that you are pleased they're comfortable enough to share it. Second, offer brief statements that say you're happy they're sharing and are receptive to hearing more. As you read the following examples, note that they focus on the fact that sharing is happening—they neither praise nor condemn (no judgment!) what is being said. They communicate that you're doing the hard work of listening to the words and attending to emotions. Note that the statements to avoid don't seem so far off the mark but subtly imply judgment.

Say This (because it keeps the conversation going)	Not That (because it passes judgment)
Tell me more.	Wow!
I'm glad I'm in your life and that I can be here for you now.	You should have come to me earlier.
It sounds like you have a lot on your mind, so I'm glad you're talking.	You seem so overwhelmed. Stop stressing out.
I appreciate that you're so open and honest with your feelings.	You care too much. It'll hurt you.
You're doing a great job of describing what happened.	If you understand what is happening this well you either should have been able to figure it out yourself or you should have come to me earlier, as soon as you understood you had a problem.

Say This (because it keeps the conversation going)	Not That (because it suggests the conversation is burdensome)
Please keep talking. I'm really interested.	Tell me everything. I need to get back to what I was doing but need to learn the whole story.
You've been through a lot. It's really healthy to talk about it.	Thanks for sharing it with me. When you hurt, I hurt.

Say This (because it keeps the conversation going)	Not That (because it feels controlling)
You have an important story to tell. I'd like to hear it.	I need to know everything going on in your life.
It means a lot to me that you feel comfortable talking to me.	I'm your parent. I'm the one you should tell it all to.

You'll know when your child is done talking. The pace of their words may slow. They may breathe more calmly, or their body language loosens. You know they're ready for guidance when they ask something like, "What would you do?"

Active listeners work hard to understand

When you express how hard you are working to understand what your child is trying to get across to you, they will experience being genuinely heard. In parallel, active listening ensures that what you are hearing is what the person is *really* saying. Start with, "This is what I heard," and then recount what they shared in your words. Then ask, "Did I understand correctly what you shared with me?" This reflection can help your child realize if they have more to say. Prompt them with, "Is there anything else you'd like to tell me to help me better understand?" Also ensure you correctly understood their emotions with, "It seems to me you are feeling. . . do I have that right?" If your child does not *yet* understand their feelings, you might facilitate their insight by saying, "When something like that happened to me, I felt like _____. Do you feel a little like that?" Children appreciate when we commit to understanding them correctly. Active listening can also include check-ins mid conversation such as, "Could you say that again? I want to be sure I understand." Or "I was with you until _____, could you explain what you meant?"

Underscoring the Benefits of Listening

This chapter started by stating the obvious: Listening is hard work. But it is so essential to you being able to guide your child today, prepare for your adolescent tomorrow, and build a lasting relationship with your child for decades to come, that I want to underscore some benefits of effective listening.

- Listening positions you to know what is going on in your child's life and therefore to support their moral development and critical thinking.
- Listening fosters independent thinking and decision-making. Answers are not given; rather, the process of seeking answers is nurtured.
- Following your model as an active and engaged listener, your child learns to collect information before drawing conclusions.
- Having learned that calm, safe spaces are places where thoughts and feelings can be processed, your child will learn to find them in the future.
- Following your model, your child will learn an essential human communication skill: respectful listening. This will prepare them for meaningful romantic relationships, friendships, and professional connections.

Your child is never too young or too old to have a story to share. One of the joys of parenting is witnessing the miracle of development. Our children's insights grow and their understanding of what surrounds them matures. The magic of listening allows you to learn how your child views the world, where their sensitivities lie, and how their capabilities to consider future implications of current actions are expanding. Equipped with this knowledge, you're ready to make your words count.

Chapter 11

Talk Wisely, Learn More

Children care deeply about what we think and want to understand our experiences and apply them to their lives. They want us to guide them to be safe, but as they grow older, they also want us to recognize that they can think for themselves. Too many adults speak *at* children, sharing wisdom and delivering warnings. We can do better. Children engage when they're spoken *with*, not talked at. When we respectfully listen and then elicit their thoughts and growing wisdom, we are positioned to guide wisely. Then our words have sticking power and our presence remains valued—meaning our adult children will want to have us around.

Preparing for Adolescence

Children need guidance. The best guidance is not just unloaded, it is offered in a way that allows children to think things through themselves so they can own the lessons. They also need to be spoken to in places they feel safe and in ways they are ready to hear. Adolescents cherish caring guidance but feel strongly about not being told what to do. Your tween or teen will seek out your words when they've learned that you are thoughtful about how they are delivered.

Shaping Your Lifelong Bond

Adults appreciate advice when it is delivered respectfully. They also cherish the stories of their elders when they convey meaningful lessons. When you set the stage in childhood for meaningful 2-way conversations and avoid the dreaded my-way-or-the-highway demands or lectures about catastrophic outcomes, you'll more likely be sitting with your adult child sharing old memories and building new ones through shared experiences.

Preparing for Conversation

What should you talk about?

What should you talk about? This is where listening pays off. Once you know what's going on, you can best offer guidance. Listening sets the tone for productive communication because emotions are revealed and the content of your children's lives unfolds. It's also how you'll earn permission to start talking. When you are understood to be someone who listens *before* jumping in, who respects your child's ability to do their own thinking, and who trusts them to handle what they can, you're more likely to be welcomed as a lifelong guide.

Sometimes you'll only be a sounding board. Other times your children need your guidance. Ask, "How can I be most helpful?" Before offering guidance, first learn what they are considering, "What do you think you might do first?" This approach frees you from always needing to have a ready-made solution. More critically, it demonstrates you see your child as the expert in their own life and solidifies your role as someone who nurtures their wisdom.

Time, spaces, and places

A great time to have a conversation is when your child is open to one. So create settings and find yourself in places where conversations might flow.

- **Feed them!** Good food makes people want to stick around for a while. It also fills our most basic needs by helping us feel safe and cared for. Being cared for makes someone open to being cared about and therefore receptive to guidance.
- **Don't start a conversation if emotions are swirling.** This might be a time to just offer comfort or to listen. Once comforted, ask them when they'd like to talk more and hear your thoughts. Book that time while they're still feeling comforted.

- **For general lessons, look for teaching opportunities.** Don't wait until your child experiences a problem you fear. Notice things while you're driving and comment on other children's behavior. Watch TV and scroll through social media together and talk about the lessons to be learned from characters' or influencers' choices. Listen to music and discuss the messages being conveyed. These conversation starters allow you to clarify values when your child is not involved. They'll listen more attentively without feeling judged and without triggering the need for your child to defend or deny their actions.

- **Some children don't want to talk while nestled in your arms.** If your child instead prefers to avoid eye contact, start conversations in the car while you're both looking forward. Or have your best conversations at night, maybe in their room when you're invited in, or while stargazing, or watching a campfire blaze. If your child does like to be hugged during conversations, that's OK too!

- **Offer privacy when tackling tough topics.** Public conversations can lead to embarrassment, an outburst, or shutting down. Private conversations show we are sensitive to their feelings and therefore those feelings will more likely be shared.

- **Texting can get conversations started.** Try, "I see something might be on your mind, I'm here for you," or, "It meant a lot that you shared _____. I'm here whenever you want me to listen more." Another great thing about text messages is that GIFs and emojis allow people to share emotions even before they're ready to say them out loud.

- **Create tech-free zones.** We worry about what being connected to a phone does to our children's ability to form critical human connections. But adults spending too much time on devices is also a problem because children need some time when we are fully present. Create a family culture where a portion of time is tech free. When devices are off, room for talking materializes.

Setting the tone for effective communication

Keep it open-ended

"How was school?" *Fine.* "Did you learn anything?" *Yes.*

If you want a productive conversation, avoid questions that can be answered with one word. Try, "Tell me what you learned in school today," or "Tell me what you think about . . ." to prime a meaningful conversation. Open-ended questions signal that we generally want to hear their thoughts, cueing them to share.

Keep it subtle

Children fear disappointing us, or worse, being rejected, and if they fear they've done something wrong, they may choose silence. For a story to unfold, sometimes you have to pass their test. Start with questions about things that matter less to help start the conversation. When you don't "freak out" about what is shared, you'll pass the test and hear more.

Keep it calm

Our brains' thinking centers do not operate very well when our emotional centers are operating at full throttle. This is true at every stage of human development from early childhood to our adult years. People think most clearly when they are calm emotionally. However, this concept is of the utmost importance during adolescence when teens often feel very fully as a typical part of development. For that reason, use cold communication as discussed in Chapter 3 to share your calm so your child, tween, or teen will get used to you being that stable, calm person they come to when they really need to think through a situation.

Keep it about how you experienced their behavior

Good conversations never begin when a person is put on the defensive. In Chapter 32, we will discuss how to remain a reliable presence throughout our child's life by having the intention and communication skill sets to rebuild trust after relationship challenges. But we can *begin* challenging conversations in a way less likely to drive us apart.

Parents have a responsibility to course correct their children. A natural way to start such a correction is to tell a child, "You did this!" Once a person feels accused, tension escalates and they may start an argument by responding, "No! You did that!" or enter denial mode: "I didn't!" Perhaps the most divisive response is if they withdraw entirely from the conversation. Instead, use the "I statement" to draw out your child's empathy and desire to make things better. It starts with, "I felt _____ when _____ happened," or "I experienced. . . ." This will bring out compassion and may lead to an apology like, "I'm sorry _____ made you feel _____. I didn't mean to. . . ."

Keep it "D" word and "G" word free

Our children's fear of disappointing us can be overwhelming. This is true even if they work hard to make you believe it's not. They feel awful when they anger or frustrate us or trouble us when they think we are burdened. Many parents use the "D" word, as in, "I'm not mad, I'm just disappointed," without understanding how deeply it can wound. Others believe guilt ("G" word) will weigh on a child's mind enough to have them behave as desired, as in, "Do you know what your behavior is doing to our family?" In fact, feelings of guilt and fears of disappointing us can weigh so heavily that our children might avoid us rather than experience the discomfort of feeling so badly.

Keep it elevated

Is our end goal as parents to have our children avoid problems? To behave well all the time? No! Our goal is for them to *thrive*. We mustn't let our conversations speak only the language of "don'ts." We must speak of potential and possibility. Even when we say, "Don't do this!" it must be because they know we believe they should live up to their potential. And any restrictions we enforce must be understood as protections put into place because of how deeply we care about and only want the best for them.

Understanding development is key to being an effective communicator

Development is a miracle. There are many rapid changes in the body, emotions, and mind on the journey to adulthood. If you understand these 3 areas of development, you'll communicate more effectively because your approach will better match your child's capabilities. Emotional development will be discussed in Chapter 12 and moral development will be discussed in Chapter 23 as the underpinning of how we raise children prepared to do and be good. In this chapter, we will discuss cognitive development, how a child's ability to think, reason, and plan matures.

Cognitive development

You cannot see cognitive development, but it changes everything in how your child relates to the world. Children and early adolescents see things concretely, exactly as they are. If you talk too much about the future or speak breathlessly about how one behavior leads to the next, they likely won't understand it. Adolescents gain the ability to think abstractly, meaning they can imagine things they can't directly see, allowing them to visualize the future and grasp the link between their actions today and consequences tomorrow. When our speech matches their cognitive capabilities, we can better help children make the connections between their actions and possible outcomes.

Getting to why and how

So often we want to understand what our children were thinking, especially when their behavior didn't make sense. So we ask, "*Why?!*" Or, we want them to think through future consequences so we ask them *how* results flow from their choices or actions. The problem with our well-intentioned questions is that many children don't yet have the planning capacities or insight to answer them. Try asking a series of *whats* instead of a lot of *whys* and *hows*. This will get you to the answers you need, using a communication strategy that matches the developmental stage of an older child or preteen. It will also help them connect actions with consequences. For example, ask, "What happened when your friend said _____ to you?" Once your child can answer what happened at that first point, then you ask, "What did your friend do after you said _____?" Follow this logic until your child has figured out for themselves the *whys* and *hows*.

Working toward that "aha!"

The lecture pushes a child to "Just get it!" before their thinking abilities enable them to do so. It is often delivered in frustration in a desperate attempt to get through to them. They hear our fear and anger but miss our intended message.

Here's the communication structure of the lecture.

Can't you see that what you're doing (Behavior A) will lead to (Consequence B)? I never imagined you being involved with (Consequence B). What is going on in that head of yours? If (Consequence B) occurs, it is likely (Consequence C) will happen to you and possibly even (Consequence D). You never would have been at risk for (Consequence B), let alone (Consequence D), if you weren't influenced by your friends. If (Consequence D) happens, I worry that (Consequences E, F, and G) could happen. Pay attention, I'm not talking just to hear myself! I'm most worried that once you and your friends are already down this path you could do (Behavior H). That can lead to (Consequence I). Do you know that a lot of people die from (Consequence I)?

What does the child hear? "Whaa whaa…a lot of them die!" They absorb our fear but can barely hear a word we're saying. Why? Because it is too abstract to consider whether current behaviors may or may not lead to imagined future outcomes. Our children and tweens don't yet have the cognitive maturity to process these thoughts. Even if they could, they can't think when they are frightened (nobody can).

We can teach the necessary lessons if we adjust how we deliver our messages. Instead of an abstract terrifying lecture, we can guide them to understand our points by presenting them calmly and slowly, one at a time. We move to the next point only after they've understood the first one. They get it . . . get it . . . get it . . . almost there . . . got it! *Aha!*

Even a panicked person can think this way. Even a school-aged child can follow ideas when presented point by point. Instead of a string of possibilities (A to B to C to D), break your thoughts into separate steps: "You are doing behavior A. What do you think might happen next? Have you thought about how B might happen? What would make B happen? What might you do to avoid it happening?" Only when your child owns the fact that their behavior could lead to B do you get them thinking about how to avoid C. The power of this communication strategy is that our children consider possible consequences step by step with their *own* ideas rather than through the lens of our fears. They'll own the lessons because they've figured them out! Our coaching helps them consider possibilities instead of relying on learning only through error. This style of guidance coaches them to listen to their inner wisdom.

Sharing Lessons Learned

Your child learns how to be a human from you. It's a sign of strength and an act of confidence to show vulnerability. Be careful, however, not to reveal what they are not yet ready to hear. Anything you discuss (or imply) could be brought up later or shape how they see you. Share judiciously, sparing details while still revealing that your lived experience has come with some emotional pain, relationship challenges, displays of unevenness, and lots of mistakes.

Disclosing your earned wisdom, and general experiences, while not sharing the details allows you to guide without the risk of oversharing. You can discuss how you've come to celebrate your strengths and learn to focus on what you do well instead of lament what you don't. You can express how your challenges came with opportunities to recover from errors and come out stronger. You can reveal that the pain you experienced in relationships likely taught you how you want to be treated and how you try to treat others. Above all, share that when you struggled, you learned to turn to people you trust for support and guidance.

CHAPTER 12

Honoring Emotional Expression Now as the Root of Lifetime Protection

Your child's lifelong relationship with their emotions is largely formed in childhood. Will they learn that their feelings are valid? Will they view vulnerability as weakness and feelings as things to be suppressed? Or will they celebrate their sensitivity? Will they recognize their own distress signals and learn to reach out to others to regain strength?

People with a rich array of emotions can have the fullest and most meaningful lives. But emotions that feel overwhelming can lead to mental health challenges such as anxiety or depression. Further, people who find it difficult to manage feelings can engage in harmful behaviors, such as drug use, to numb their thoughts or suppress their feelings.

As parents, we want our children to benefit from the richness and depth of their feelings while also learning to manage emotional discomfort in ways that strengthen them. We first commit to standing by our children through their emotional highs and lows by giving them the safe space to learn how feelings affect their mood and behavior. Then, we support them to develop skills to manage those feelings comfortably and healthfully.

Preparing for Adolescence

Emotional health is not about always feeling happy or even content. It is about having real emotions in response to actual situations and managing them well. When we support our children to comfortably experience a range of emotions, they'll more confidently share the breadth and intensity of their feelings with us during adolescence.

Shaping Your Lifelong Bond

Believing they should be able to handle whatever comes their way, many people deny their emotions rather than seeking human support to help manage them. When we raise our children to have a healthy relationship with their emotions, they'll more likely see us as safe people with whom they can share the complexities of their lives. Emotional support is at the root of long-standing healthy mutual reliance.

Naming an Uncomfortable Truth

I don't know how your own childhood experiences formed your relationship with emotions. But I do know you're committed to doing what is right for your child because you're reading a book about being an effective, engaged, and loving parent. *And* I know that our children need us to hear them and to help them learn to manage life when it doesn't feel good. But *becoming comfortable with their discomfort is uncomfortable.* Why? Let's name 2 reasons. The first is that we care so deeply about them that their pain is harder to bear than our own. The second reason is harder to discuss but must be named. Many of us simply don't have the vocabulary or muscle memory to help children manage distress because our own feelings were not attended to when we were young. Since we turned out "OK," we may worry we will spoil or make them more vulnerable if we allow them the room to feel their feelings fully. Before we move on, I assure you that love *never* spoils a child, it only makes them more secure and prepared to pass along that security to the next generation.

Before you read some words that might serve as unpleasant reminders of what you may have heard as a child, ask yourself a critical question. Even if you are resilient and turned out "OK," is OK *really* good enough for you? Is it good enough for your child? If the following applies to you, some space for reflection might help you give your child's emotional life the full attention that it deserves. If it does not apply to you, it may be worth reading because it likely applies to someone you care about.

Some of us growing up may have received spoken and unspoken messages that being good meant being silent about our feelings. "Boys don't cry. Girls shouldn't complain. Big kids don't whine." Some of us had our feelings actively belittled. "You don't see me complaining, do you? You're a kid! You don't have real problems. You're making a big deal of nothing." Some were told we were responsible for our own pain. "Well, sure you're going to get teased if you act like _____." Or, "How would you expect your father to act if you've made him so angry?" In the worst-case scenario, you may have learned that expressed feelings led to abusive remarks or physical harm.

It is difficult to be attentive to others' emotions when we have learned to suppress our own. Reading about why it matters may motivate you to parent differently than you were parented, but it is hardly enough. There is a lingering and deeply ingrained impact left by how our emotional lives were regarded when we were children. That's the point. Ask yourself if you can be even stronger and more content with yourself if there isn't shame associated with your feelings. The first step of breaking the cycle is choosing to behave differently. Although your first impulse may be to replay the scripts spoken to you or to choose to avoid emotions, you can change that. You may find that reflection with others or professional support is helpful.

Your feelings are showing

Before you read on to consider suggestions on what words you might use in supporting your child to have a healthy relationship with their emotions, I want to underscore that it is what you *don't say* that may send the loudest messages. If emotions make you uncomfortable and you leave the room, furrow your brow, or cross your arms when your child is experiencing their feelings, they will learn they should withhold their feelings in your presence. They may do so to avoid your judgment, or because they choose to spare you any discomfort that they intuitively learn is more than you can handle. In either case, your unspoken reactions can limit your power as a source of security and safety because your child may not turn to you when you are most needed. They also may learn that they too should avoid their feelings.

Modeling

Showing up for our children begins by modeling. Through our actions they learn how to prepare for adulthood including how to experience joys and deal with pain and frustrations. Modeling is always important, but in this case, the intentional effort you put into modeling emotional health might do you a great deal of good. We easily fall into patterns we might assume are inalterable, believing it is our destiny to be silent or even suffer. Knowing you are modeling for your child forces you to notice those patterns and motivates you to do better for yourself. Intentionality is about pausing when something doesn't feel right and asking yourself, "Now that my child is watching, how can I demonstrate seeking support and engaging in self-care?"

Do This	Not That
Show up. Stand by your child. Listen without judgment.	Walk out of the room in discomfort. Say things that suggest emotions are wrong or more than you can handle. Ignore the expression of strong emotions assuming (or hoping) they'll go away.

Say This	Not That
I've got a lot on my mind, but nothing is more important than you.	You're upsetting me. I have my own problems to deal with.
I don't know quite the right thing to say now. But I'm here with you; you're not alone.	I don't know what to do for you. No words I say seem to come out right.
You are full of feelings. It is healthy to be the kind of person who has lots of emotions.	You are too emotional.
I know you are hurting. What can I do to support you?	You are being too dramatic; just get over it. You are making a big deal over nothing.
It's great that you're letting out your feelings.	You don't have to cry about it. Calm down.
Thank you for coming to me to tell me how you feel.	I'm too busy. (This can be said through words or actions like choosing distance.)
One of the best things about you is how sensitive you are.	You need to toughen up; life can be hard.
Feelings can be uncomfortable and sometimes you'll learn to manage the fullness of your emotions. I'm going to support you to get there and to find you the professional support you deserve (see Chapter 22).	You need help. (The word "help" could come off as judgmental or condescending and implies someone else needs to do it for you. The phrase "support you deserve" suggests that you can get past this with a professional "supporting" your abilities.)

Supporting Emotional Development

We must raise children to understand no emotion is wrong, but some are uncomfortable and need to be managed or addressed. This removes judgment and creates room to learn how to accept a range of emotions. Few of us have problems accepting joy, so let's focus on emotions that upset us. Suppressed emotions can delay the pain and ultimately end up being released in harmful ways. They also may engender shame or self-hatred which can lead to depression or leave us unsettled and anxious.

If you are blessed with a child with a full range of feelings, celebrate that your child can feel fully because that predicts they will get the most out of life, meaningfully connect with others, and ultimately gain the deep satisfaction that comes from knowing they matter to others. The downside to feeling so fully is that they will possess distressing feelings. Your goal is to support your child to notice and manage those feelings in a way that enables them to flourish by developing their own muscle memory to manage life's complexities.

If their response is "wha-a-at?" and "who cares?"

Often young people with rich inner lives, deep sensitivity, and endless compassion work hard to not let any of that show. If you are duped by this feigned indifference, you'll lose the opportunity to help your child grow into their feelings. Remember this: it's harder to say, "I care so much it hurts," than it is to say, "It doesn't matter." If a child or teen wants to avoid a tough conversation or ignore a stress-inducing circumstance, it is easier to put on earphones and say, "Wha-a-at?" or question "About what? I wasn't listening." Your child needs you to not take their response at face value. You might say, "I know you're disappointed/angry/frustrated right now. It's OK to tuck away feelings for a while. Sometimes I do that until I'm ready to deal with how I feel. We'll talk later about how to make this situation better." If your child acts like they don't even notice what is going on, they may be signaling that dealing with an issue head-on and face-to-face is not their preferred approach. Take a drive and start a conversation while you can avoid eye contact. Or offer guidance in general terms by commenting on something you know many young people worry about. Then tell them you'll feel better if you give them advice in case that ever becomes an issue for them. You can also take advantage of one of the greatest strengths of childhood and adolescence: how much they care about and want to protect their friends. As a doctor, I often give advice by speaking to young people about what they should know in case a friend ever comes to them in need. This approach is always well received.

Healthy emotional management

We can take 2 very different approaches to manage uncomfortable or intense feelings. Either approach can be appropriate depending on circumstances and therefore our children should be skilled in both practices. One strategy helps us escape feelings, and the other helps deal with them.

Escape as emotional management

Escaping is not the same as ignoring. Rather, we choose to give ourselves a break, an "instant vacation" from our feelings. Sometimes we'll return to them and sometimes we'll move on so we can preserve our energy to deal with more pressing concerns. We should choose vacations that don't allow our thoughts and worries to intrude into them. Reading a book is one of the best vacations. We imagine the sights, sounds, and smells. We experience feelings as we immerse ourselves into the story, leaving no room for our problems to intrude. Mindfulness activities such as meditation or yoga can also prevent intrusive thoughts as our focus on the present allows neither memories from the past nor worries about the future to disturb us.

Helping your child learn to escape in a healthy way may serve as drug prevention. Substance use disorder can start as an effort to escape stressful thoughts or tough emotions, but the escape substances offer is temporary and extremely dangerous. An "instant vacation" is a much better, healthier strategy.

Dealing with emotions directly

There are many healthy ways to directly manage emotions. First, we can bring awareness to the issues driving our emotions and, when possible, address those issues. Second, we can join with other people to gain strength knowing that in time we will lend our strength to others. Lastly, we can name our emotions as a first step of controlling them rather than being controlled by them. Once named, we can focus on expressing them in a productive manner, so they do not build up over time.

Name and express thoughts and feelings

Many people place stressful emotions into figurative containers hoping they'll deal with those feelings later. The problem is that life continues to offer challenges, and feelings added to the container eventually build up. The walls of the container need to become stronger to hold them all in. When the walls become strong enough to hold a lot of our burdens, we can't penetrate them to access what is stored within them. When we cannot connect with our feelings, we become numb. Especially for sensitive people, that can feel worse than being stressed.

Safe containers enable us to function. But they must be opened at some point, or the feelings inside may come out in ways we cannot control. We help our children build emotional intelligence when they learn to name their feelings and create safe spaces to express them. Naming them is as a first step to dealing with them. "I'm feeling angry/confused/frustrated/hurt or sad." Processing emotions may be harder than naming them. We can support our children to express stressful or emotional experiences in a way that works for them. We want them to be able to say to themselves, "This hurts, but I can _____ it out." Each person's journey is to learn what strategy best fits them.

- *I can write it out.* Writing allows us to let go of emotions while clarifying and organizing them. Journaling creates a safe, private space to express feelings.
- *I can talk it out.* Like writing, this allows the feelings to be released. Being genuinely listened to while sharing thoughts and feelings reinforces that we all matter.
- *I can pray it out.* Being connected to something bigger than us serves as a reminder of the greater meaning of our lives. It can allow those who pray to hand over their burdens.
- *I can laugh it out.* Laughing creates a reset—a chance to start over. My grandmother, Belle Moore, taught me that people with a sense of humor can survive almost anything. *What kernels of wisdom about managing distress were passed on to you from your elders?*
- *I can cry it out.* Tears are nature's way of letting go of our feelings and telling others something is going on for us. Tears can express joy, pain, or grief. Sobbing offers a deep release that can also reset our mood.
- *I can dance/sing/rap/sculpt/draw it out.* Some people may find creative expression easier and more powerful than finding words to communicate and release their feelings.

89

- *I can scream it out!* Screaming can release our raw emotions. To make it safe, we can teach our children to scream into a pillow or find a secluded place to release their deepest feelings.

Avoid messages that restrict how children *should* react or feel

Too many boys have been raised to bury their feelings and tough it out and too many girls have been told they must always be kind and selfless. These gender-based messages can leave people disconnected from their feelings and aspirations. Strong men address feelings, are sensitive to the needs of their partners, and are engaged fathers, brothers, sons, and friends. Young women should display sensitivity, as we all should, but not at their own expense. Self-advocacy is not selfishness and assertiveness is not aggression.

All children regardless of gender identity need to hear the following statements:

- People gain strength from each other. Form meaningful relationships in which you both draw and lend strength.
- It is brave and responsible to talk about your emotions.
- Parents should be affectionate with their children and tell them how much they are loved.
- We all suffer at times; we don't need to be alone when we do.
- I am proud when you share how you feel, especially when you are clear about what you need.
- I appreciate your thoughts and feelings and I'm proud you can state them clearly.

The emotional brilliance of teens

Teens' emotions develop at a remarkable pace. They read feelings voraciously, quickly learn to judge others' intentions, and become increasingly aware of how they make others feel. This explains much of the exuberance of adolescence because they feed on others' joy which contributes to their desire to spend so much time around peers. In parallel, supporting their peers through challenging moments becomes a driving force of teen culture. However, their incredible sensitivity can also cause them to overanalyze or assume others unspoken thoughts (ie, "Why are you looking at me like that?!") or to feel emotionally overloaded.

This is a typical part of development as the parts of the brain that process emotions develop rapidly during adolescence, but there is not *yet* enough life experience to determine how they might interpret these emotional inputs. The parts of their brains that think through situations will catch up and their life experience will be earned. In the meantime, caring adults' calming presence helps to settle them, if and when they are on emotional overdrive (see Chapter 3). Knowing this also helps us understand why we need to be clear in our communication. Uncertainty drives anxiety and leaves our intentions open to misinterpretation. When we state the whys behind our behaviors, we eliminate uncertainty. For example, "I set this rule because I care about your safety and when you did _____ it placed you in danger."

Honoring Your Child's Emotions Is the Root of a Lifelong Relationship

Lighthouse Parenting is a framework for parenting now that pays off by strengthening your lifelong relationship. When your child sees you as a source of comfort, they'll turn to you for decades to come. The inspirational truth is that you will also be able to lean into your adult child as a source of your own comfort. Perhaps even more profound, if you are a source of validation for them because you see the best in them and allow them, without judgment, to feel what they need to feel, they will forever see you as the person who helped them discover their innate sense of value and self-worth.

CHAPTER 13

Parenting Neurodivergent Children

Dr Eric Flake was invited to contribute this chapter. Dr Flake is a developmental and behavioral pediatrician and is also a retired colonel. For the past 25 years, he led efforts within the Department of Defense ensuring families serving our nation with neurodivergent children received the support services they deserved to enable their children to thrive while the service member parent could defend our country.

Parenting a neurodivergent child comes with unique challenges and rewards. It's a journey that requires a delicate balance of unconditional love and high but realistic expectations, where you nurture your child's growth while celebrating their uniqueness.

Over the years, parents have asked me critically important questions about parenting a neurodivergent child with individual and special needs, including

- Do the principles of effective parenting apply to all children, including those with special needs?
- How do I know if I am causing more stress on them by setting high expectations or setting specific progress goals?
- Do I have unrealistic expectations for their growth due to existing or emerging developmental or behavioral challenges?
- How do I know if their behavior results from their developmental challenges, or is it a part of typical childhood, or the changes that accompany adolescence?

As you can imagine, these are difficult questions to answer. Let's start by saying that the core principles of effective parenting work for ALL children. Still, there may be cases in which we adjust our communication approach for those who are neurodivergent or have a neurodevelopmental condition. Children have unique needs, and my advice here will be general; often, children deserve a team of professionals to tailor the best strategies to support them.

Neurodivergence and Neurodevelopmental Disorders

Neurodivergent individuals follow unique developmental pathways and may require additional support and attention because of a developmental issue. A child following a typical developmental path is referred to as neurotypical.

Neurodivergent children may have conditions such as autism spectrum disorder (ASD), attention-deficit/hyperactivity disorder (ADHD), intellectual or learning disabilities, sensory processing or behavior regulation difficulties, anxiety or depression, and more. We estimate from past research that at least one-third of all youth experience a neurodivergent pathway.

Neurodiversity is a term widely accepted to help understand neurological differences and emphasize human variation as a child progresses on their individual developmental journey. We celebrate divergence and appreciate systems of support that work to intentionally embrace neurodiversity into school and community systems. Parenting a neurodivergent child can add additional and unanticipated layers of complexity to the rewarding and challenging journey of parenting.

Communication Challenges for Children With Social Thinking Differences

A major social developmental milestone is recognizing that others may have different thoughts and feelings than our own. This key development of social communication begins in the toddler years and continues to mature into adulthood. However, some neurodivergent children may have more difficulty developing an understanding that other people have different thoughts, feelings, and beliefs than those they hold. This limitation of perception is often referred to as having challenges with theory of mind. New insight highlights that this is a common challenge for neurodivergent individuals, particularly those with neurodevelopmental disorders such as ASD and some with ADHD.

Divergence in the theory of mind is one of the principal characteristics that lead to being identified as autistic. Individuals with ADHD *may* also demonstrate challenges with communication because they may prefer to overfocus on an area of interest and/or they may have difficulty focusing depending on the subject matter. For example, a child with ADHD might notice so many things in their physical environment that they have trouble focusing on a task. In contrast, they may be able to hyper- or overfocus on a task that is in their strength area, such as communicating deeply with a person or diving into video games. This variability of focus has proven to result in either an advanced or underdeveloped social awareness or theory of mind for some children with ADHD. Parents of a neurodivergent child know their child's neurodevelopmental disability and likely know best which of the points in this chapter apply to them and in which areas they might already be gifted.

Neurodivergent children and youth may have difficulties understanding the intentions of others by looking at their gestures and listening to their words. This makes it difficult for them to anticipate behaviors or actions likely to happen next. These limitations in insight, the ability to look inside another to determine their mood, feelings, and thoughts, can be challenging and, at times, provoke unwanted behaviors or responses. This difficulty in interpreting others' communication signals also leads to social and communication challenges. Furthermore, these challenges may impact a child's ability to improve their social skills as they will find it harder to absorb lessons from social communication successes and missteps. Often increased stress and anxiety emerge as it is difficult for neurodiverse children to fully determine what is happening around them and to anticipate what may happen next. It is at this point when parents often feel frustrated and question themselves; they may be using effective parenting and communication principles, yet their child doesn't respond like experts suggest they will. Developing insight (or an inside sight) is a valuable learned skill that for some individuals will require more time and intentional instruction.

The benefit of looking at a child's level of insight is to help parents and loved ones understand that neurodivergent children often struggle with understanding the mental thoughts of others. There are 2 critical points for parents to know to better assess their children's behaviors. First, limitations in insight can help explain why, at times, when a parent is communicating a message or instruction, the message doesn't seem to connect with their child. It is *not* defiance or a willful effort to ignore the parent's guidance. Second, difficulty attending to or interpreting other people's thoughts and feelings can limit a child's understanding of the vast array of emotions and nonverbal communications. This does *not* mean an individual with difficulty interpreting or perceiving what is happening around them lacks empathy.

One way to understand this concept better is to imagine that a neurodivergent child may have challenges with their social vision and, as such, they benefit from additional training just as a pair of glasses are utilized to help clarify the vision of someone who has trouble seeing. Finding the correct glasses would not change their sight entirely but would offer a tool to help their vision. The tools to help with social vision may assist a neurodivergent individual to work and play better with neurotypical people as they learn social communication strategies from each other. The goal is to seek together the right prescription or supports so your neurodivergent child can better "read" the environment.

Key Communication Challenges in Neurodivergent Youth

As parents embark on raising children and adolescents with communication and connection challenges, understanding the unique obstacles they may face is crucial to decreasing their frustration and empowering them with productive actions. Neurodivergent individuals, particularly those with social thinking differences, often encounter difficulties interpreting and responding effectively to social cues. The challenges they experience include

1. Perspective Taking: Neurodivergent individuals may find it challenging to understand others' nonverbal cues such as thoughts, feelings, and intentions, which can lead to conversational difficulties.

2. Literal Interpretation: Sarcasm, humor, and metaphors may be misunderstood, leading to miscommunication and social awkwardness.

3. Flexibility: Rigidity in thinking can hinder a neurodivergent child from responding to subtle communication signals. The child may struggle to adjust their communication style based on the situation or the clues another person is giving as to what they need or expect.

4. Impulsivity and Blurting: Some children may impulsively share their thoughts without understanding that they need to take turns speaking or acting before considering the impact on others. This can lead to social challenges and misunderstandings.

Supporting Social Communication in Neurodivergent Children

A child's neurodevelopmental task of learning to "read the room," including understanding spoken and unspoken cues, can be made easier by the development of theory of mind skills. Parents can support their child in the development of these skills by applying effective parenting principles. Providing your child with opportunities to interact with other children and adults will help them learn about different perspectives and see how their thoughts and feelings differ from those of others.

I will draw from the core principles of Lighthouse Parenting to underscore effective parenting for a neurodivergent child. It begins with using a balanced parenting style that involves cultivating an environment where both love and expectation coexist harmoniously. It means showering your child with acceptance and understanding while also setting appropriate expectations that challenge them to reach their fullest potential. For children with autism, this balance is crucial. Love provides the foundation of emotional security, while expectation fuels personal growth. When these elements are in harmony, your child feels valued for who they are and encouraged to explore their capabilities.

The next step is to determine an action plan for impact. Creating an effective action plan begins with understanding your child's strengths, challenges, and needs. This information can be assisted by asking other caring professionals, family, and friends who know your child. Tailor your approach to suit your child's unique profile and establish realistic expectations for their next steps of development. Prioritize stability, security, and safety within your home environment. Establish routines and create sensory-friendly spaces that help your child feel comfortable. Setting achievable goals aligned with their developmental stage will allow them to experience success and build confidence. This is followed by periodic review and adjustments to the plan as your child grows and changes.

The Path of a Lighthouse Parent With Neurodivergent Children

Let us consider how applying the core principles of Lighthouse Parenting will assist your neurodivergent child in optimizing their growth and development.

Build relationship: offer stability, security, safety

Building a strong parent-child relationship involves providing stability, security, and safety. Consistency in routines and clear communication helps your child feel secure. Creating an environment where they can express themselves without fear of judgment is necessary for them to be able to communicate their needs. Offering support during challenging moments allows them to understand that trust is a cornerstone of your relationship. Your child will be more open and ready for growth and influence when trust is established.

Modeling and knowing

Children, especially those with autism, often learn by observing and practicing. Model the behavior, values, and emotional regulation (see Chapter 3) you want them to adopt. In addition, they can practice using 3 strategies.

- Role-playing by pretending and practicing a desired behavior.
- Video modeling, in which a behavior is watched with the intent for it to be imitated in the future.
- Reviewing social stories, which can provide specific information about what to expect in a future situation and why. Social stories do this by offering short descriptions of a future experience introduced through a set of pictures which allow discussion of potential events without any of the real-life pressures.

These techniques can be powerful when used individually or in combination and have been shown to be effective ways to help teach expected behavior and help neurodivergent children understand emotions.

To further develop theory of mind skills, use these techniques to express thoughts and share feelings in a safe, secure environment. Learning critical skills such as listening and taking turns talking can be done by practice through playing and modeling.

Practice and modeling will help your child feel more comfortable as they experience various, often difficult-to-understand, emotions. Emotional picture cards can often help teach a wide array of emotions and can even be used to illustrate that one can experience multiple emotions simultaneously. Read stories about feelings and talk to/with your child about them. Stories about emotions can help children to learn about different emotions and how they are expressed. Watch movies and TV shows about emotions to illustrate examples of characters' thoughts and feelings. This is more effective if discussion regarding the nuances of each scenario follows.

Be patient and give your child time to understand and learn. Measure their progress not by what society suggests is "normal" but against their individual journey. Celebrate even small achievements that contribute to their overall development. Critically, root your unconditional love for them in the strengths they possess.

Building trust

Your efforts to communicate with your neurodivergent child in a way that they both understand and are comfortable with earns their trust in you. It creates an atmosphere where they feel safe expressing their thoughts and emotions without fear of rejection. It is important to respect that, at times, they may need personal space and time if they become overwhelmed. Figure out what triggers your child or gets them upset so that you can assist them before they or you get overwhelmed. They might find sounds, smells, tastes, or textures objectionable or comforting. One way of understanding this is that they receive communication signals from these other senses that neurotypical people ignore. Because of this, effective, safe, and trustworthy communication from you begins with respecting their need for different sensory inputs and learning what provides them with sensory comfort.

Protection: resilience and thriving

While protection is essential, fostering resilience is equally important. Shielding your child from all challenges won't equip them to navigate the world. Children with neurodevelopmental challenges can learn coping strategies and problem-solving skills and communicate what is needed for personal resilience.

Ongoing encouragement to gradually step out of their comfort zone and celebrate their resilience and growth will result in them thriving.

Preparation: self-advocacy

As your child grows, empower them with self-advocacy skills. Teach them about their neurodivergence, strengths, and challenges. You can highlight their strengths and then empower your child to help others recognize that neurodiverse people uniquely contribute to both small- and large-group settings. Learning to embrace one's neurodiversity will allow them to utilize language that expresses their needs to others and fosters independence. Parental preparation includes equipping yourself with knowledge about the strengths of neurodiversity found in individuals with neurodevelopmental conditions such as autism. Learning about available resources ensures you can advocate effectively on their behalf.

Reliability: rules

Maintain consistency in your interactions and expectations. Children who like to think in black-and-white, concrete concepts struggle with gray scenarios but often thrive in predictable environments. Clearly defining rules and expectations and offering them a sense of structure can be critical. Picture schedules, timers, daily planning, and rehearsing can often minimize anxiety and help with clear expectations. Essential to social interaction is learning that there are rules and orders to communicating. Learning and teaching these rules is critical to help provide structure. However, as a Lighthouse Parent, it is also important to anticipate that flexibility is important to accommodate your child's unique needs and challenges. Flexibility does not imply doing away with the structure. Rather, it means that it may take more time for your child to benefit from the structure, or you may need to find a different way to explain the reason the rules exist.

Wisely Communicating Important Messages to Your Child

Say This (about your child's strengths and limitations)	Not That	Because
I love your unique perspective on life.	Why can't you be like everyone else?	This allows a child to recognize that their unique combination of strengths and challenges provides a diversity that benefits those around them.
You are really good at [specific skills].	Why are you always so [negative adjective]?	Looking at a child's strengths can have a long-lasting impact on how they see themselves, resulting in improved behavior because of their desire to meet expectations.

Say This (when engaging your child's thoughtfulness)	Not That	Because
I believe you. Your feelings are important to me.	It is all in your head.	Validating thoughts and feelings and allowing them to be explored in a safe and secure environment minimizes stress and anxiety and results in a child being receptive to achieving new developmental milestones.
You appear to be in tune with lots of thoughts and feelings. I see that you are upset right now.	You're too sensitive. Stop crying!	Neurodivergent individuals often feel and think at profound levels and experience their senses in ways others may never even know possible. This can be overwhelming at times and a source of valuable perspective.

Say This (about performance)	Not That	Because
I am proud of you for sticking with this. It shows a lot of courage. You haven't accomplished your goal yet, but you can if you keep learning and growing.	You will never change.	Viewing the courage demonstrated by children who have additional life challenges empowers them to have hope for future endeavors and minimizes demoralization. Encouraging the growth mindset will be discussed in Chapter 25. Use the power of the word "yet."
How about you try _____?	Don't do _____.	All children benefit by being guided toward what they can do instead of being told what they cannot do. This may be particularly important for a neurodivergent child to overcome limitations by building on and expanding existing strengths.
We need people in this world who see it differently. I appreciate the way you think about/ do things. You are a great example of a self-advocate.	You will grow out of it.	We must value diversity in all aspects of our culture. Accepting neurodivergence has allowed individuals to come forward and helps us better understand their uniqueness and potential contributions. This also minimizes the shame or stigma associated with feeling different.
You are valued for who you are, and I admire who you are becoming.	I couldn't tell that you were different.	Telling someone, "I can't see your difference," is well intentioned but implies it is something better to be hidden. Valuing someone for their unique contributions instead of complimenting them on their ability to conform to norms will continue to empower them to meet their optimal developmental pathway.

A Lighthouse Parent Can Be the Right Guide for a Neurodivergent Child

Parenting children and adolescents with various degrees of communication and connection challenges requires dedication and adaptability. By being aware of the unique communication obstacles neurodivergent individuals may face and by implementing effective strategies to foster communication, emotional connections, and social skills, parents can create a nurturing and supportive environment for their children to flourish. The insight you develop into your child's neurodivergence will empower you with the knowledge to establish appropriate and realistic expectations for measured growth and development.

We started with a commonly asked question: "How do I know if their behavior results from their developmental challenges, or is it a part of typical childhood or the changes that accompany adolescence?" The answer is that your child will have all of the expected challenges of a typical child or adolescent *and* have the unique stressors of learning to improve their ability to read people. With your guidance, meeting that challenge will be far easier.

Parenting a neurodivergent child is a journey filled with learning and love. Embracing this journey with compassion and understanding allows parents to guide their children toward developing meaningful relationships with others. To be clear, your child needs compassion and understanding. So do you. This journey can be simultaneously fulfilling and frustrating. It can be challenging to parent a child whose communication "wiring" may differ significantly from your own. However, by approaching the journey with empathy, patience, and flexibility, you can create a nurturing environment that allows your child to flourish and reach their full potential.

Tips for Lighthouse Parenting a Neurodivergent Child

1. Unconditional Love: The power of unconditional love should never be understated and can be the foundation of all your actions. Remain committed to seeing your child's abundant strengths.

2. Educate Yourself: Learn about your child's specific neurodivergent disability, whether it's autism, ADHD, dyslexia, or any other condition. Understand their strengths, challenges, and how their challenges impact development.

3. Embrace Acceptance: Accept your child, neurodivergence and all. Celebrate differences and empower them to embrace their identity and acknowledge their challenges while at the same time not expecting them to conform to what society calls typical.

4. Open Communication: Create an open and judgment-free space for your child to express themselves. Encourage discussion about feelings and emotions, sharing experiences and challenges, and listening actively without interrupting.

5. Individualized Approach: Recognize that each neurodivergent child is unique. What works for your child might not work for another.

6. Sensory Sensitivities: Be mindful of sensory sensitivities. Create a sensory-friendly environment to help your child feel more comfortable and reduce sensory overload.

7. Predictable Routine: Neurodivergent children often thrive on predictability. Visual schedules and clear, consistent routines can help reduce anxiety and create a sense of stability.

8. Positive Reinforcement: Use positive reinforcement and rewards to encourage desired behaviors. Celebrate their accomplishments, no matter how small, and focus on strengths.

9. Patience and Flexibility: Practice patience as you navigate challenges together. Be creative, flexible, and resourceful in your expectations and approaches, adapting them as needed. If something isn't working, talk to other parents about how they've managed a similar issue. Ideally, problem-solve with your child so they can guide you on how flexibility in meeting their needs will pay off.

10. Advocate for Your Child: Maintain a team of schools, health care professionals, and other caregivers to advocate for your child to receive appropriate support and accommodations.

11. Encourage Independence: Promote independence by teaching age-appropriate life skills. Encourage them to make choices and decisions, fostering confidence and self-reliance.

12. Simplify Tasks: Break tasks into smaller steps, and use visual aids (social stories, daily checklist) if necessary.

13. Foster Social Skills: Help your child develop social skills through social groups and therapy, if needed. Seek peer support via clubs, organizations, or support groups that cater to your child's interests and needs and/or are a supportive social environment for neurodivergent individuals. Help nurture the development of their theory of mind. This will involve helping them build empathy, learn the importance of sharing and taking turns, and develop the skills to read social cues.

14. Manage Transitions: Changes can be challenging; visual cues, timers, and warnings help them prepare for transitions between activities or environments.

15. Celebrate Progress: Focus on progress rather than comparing against others. Celebrate even small achievements and milestones, and recognize your child's efforts in their growth.

Part 4

Protection

I choose to be a Lighthouse Parent . . . I'll look down at the rocks to be sure they don't crash against them.

CHAPTER 14

Hovering Drives Children Away: Preparation Is the Best Protection

It is our duty and joy to protect our infants who are born vulnerable and defenseless and our young children who are wired to explore but have no sense of limits. Our older children don't depend on us for basic survival needs but continue to need our protection in the form of monitoring to remain within safe boundaries. Our instinct to protect our children is so deeply embedded that no matter their age, we still wish we could wrap them in bubble wrap. Our challenge is that our children, no matter their age, should explore as much of the world as they can handle and need us to encourage them to stretch into new territory.

When efforts to shield children from harm cross the line into overprotection, the message we send is, "I don't trust you." If you inadvertently send this message of mistrust, it will undermine your child's growing confidence because they'll question if they should trust themselves. Further, when we are overprotective, we send the message that we see them as fragile rather than resilient. Knowing you see them as fragile, they may grow to see themselves as easily broken.

Lighthouse Parents communicate that our goal is to prepare our children to make their own wise decisions and learn to protect themselves. Central to our role as guides is that our children learn to trust themselves when we trust them. We can more genuinely trust them with independent decision-making when we have adequately prepared them to navigate life's important decisions and challenges.

Preparing for Adolescence

Adolescents have a need to explore new horizons. They want guidance and protection but only when they feel they need it. If you are overprotective during their childhood, your tween or teen may resent your protective instincts and hide their growing independence from you, rather than risk you limiting their experiences.

Shaping Your Lifelong Bond

Interdependence works best when each individual could function on their own but chooses to invite another person into their life. If your adult child views you as a hovering parent, they'll never trust that you will honor their independent thoughts and decisions and therefore may not choose to include you in the details of their life.

Preparation *Is* Long-term Protection

Let's start off with a shared understanding of the critical nature of protection. Lighthouse Parents do and must be protective when necessary. *"I'll look down at the rocks to be sure they don't crash against them . . ."* But they also know that it is only through their trust that their children will begin assuming responsibility for their own safety and for the steps they need to be successful. *"I'll look into the waves and trust they'll learn to ride them . . ."* They also understand that children need guidance to build their own skills and therefore remain *"committed to prepare them to do so."* Critically, they also recognize that life will throw each of us curveballs and children, of every age, can sometimes need the safety and guidance a parent best offers. *"I'll remain a source of light they can seek whenever they need a safe and secure return."*

So how do we offer real protection? First, we draw from our protective instincts and respond quickly and unapologetically when there is real danger. We discuss this more in the next chapter. But short of a true threat, the best strategy is to offer the balance between protection and guidance, while trusting our child's capacity to gain wisdom from life's lessons. We protect them best when we help our children process their experiences to ultimately learn to make good decisions and choose their own safe paths. When we get this balance right, we can more confidently (I didn't say easily 😊) let them approach new experiences, knowing they possess skillsets and thinking abilities that will enable them to successfully navigate both good and challenging times.

Preparation is at the heart of this book

Protection and preparation are tightly intertwined. All the chapters in Part 5 on building resilience are about preparing your child to flourish even when life is tough. And Chapters 23 through 27 are about helping your child develop the character strengths known to prepare them to thrive. Part 6 explores specific strategies to prepare your child to productively process life experiences to determine how to safely stretch their limits. It also guides you on how to prepare them with communication strategies that will empower them to follow their own values even when exposed to real-life pressures or manipulation in digital spaces.

Getting past your need to hover

I suspect that if we kept the discussion at that idealized place in which none of us actually lives, most parents would agree that overprotection sends the wrong message to children. But it is sometimes difficult to restrain from jumping in when real life presents itself. Why do we so easily go into protective mode when there is no actual danger? Why do we overmanage our children's lives when there is a part of us that understands it may be interfering with them learning to make their own decisions? My guess is that if your tendency is to hover, you've earned the right to feel you must be highly protective. Reflecting on what drives your need to jump in is the first step in being able to consider that your child may be more protected when you focus on preparing them instead of doing it all for them.

The following are some scenarios in which parents overmanage their children's lives followed by the reasons parents have shared with me on why they struggle with standing on the sidelines. Read on and see if any of their thoughts apply to you. If not, they might apply to someone else in your child's life. I've also offered some thoughts in each scenario on why greater independence will benefit your child in the hopes of allowing you to pause to reframe your thinking. However, because your own experiences likely drive your protective nature, expect stepwise progress. You might start by standing a bit more on the sidelines as you observe that when your child is given the opportunity to manage more of their own life—still under your caring and watchful gaze—they gain confidence.

Some parents go into protective mode even when there is no danger. If this describes you, what might be driving your need to be overprotective?

- You may not have been watched closely enough as a child. Perhaps you experienced real dangers because your caregivers were unaware of something happening to you or of risks you were experiencing? If this is the case, you may be naturally inclined to believe you must know everything in your child's life. Rest assured that Chapter 15 is about protecting your child from real dangers. And, as a Lighthouse Parent, you'll have the kind of open communication that will make it more likely that your child will come to you when they need your guidance or protection.

- You may see highly protective parents who seem to offer their children every opportunity. Possibly, you resent that you were given so much range to create your own opportunities. Perhaps you feel you would be more successful if your parents had showered you with more opportunities. If so, you might lean toward overmanaging your child's activities. Trust that your child's best chance of finding what gives them the most meaning and satisfaction is having the ability to select some of their own opportunities based on their focused interests and burgeoning talents.

Some parents too easily go into fix-it mode when their child makes a mistake. Might you have difficulty watching your child learn from life's lessons?

- Do you tend to go into catastrophic thinking? If so, when your child experiences a mistake, do you assume that is the beginning of a series of failures? If you believe mistakes inevitably lead to catastrophic failures, you would be justified in trying to prevent them. I invite you to consider that many initial failures create opportunities to do better the next time. Failures are the way we learn to grow and to understand our strengths and limitations. Therefore, protecting a child from all failures harms them by limiting their growth.

Some parents unnecessarily manage the details of their child's life to avoid something that makes the parents themselves anxious (like a bad grade or an uncomfortable social interaction). Might you be reliving your childhood through your child's experiences?

- Do your child's social struggles give you anxiety? Is this because it's hard to imagine them uncomfortable? Or might it be that you had discomfort growing up and want to make sure your child does not experience the same pain? Remember that developing social skills will contribute to their thriving and that being temporarily boosted through you solving a problem will not prepare them with the skillsets they need.
- Have you fallen victim to the belief that the college your child is accepted into or their first job will determine their life? If so, you likely feel as though you are parenting on a treadmill and if you don't keep up, your child will be left behind. If so, please return as often as needed to Chapter 2, where we discussed setting the right goals. Here is a brief recap.
  - Goal 1: Commit to having open communication within your family.
  - Goal 2: Prepare each child to navigate the world independently but to simultaneously know the importance of relying on others.
  - Goal 3: Raise your child to be well prepared to get a second job.
  - Goal 4: Commit to raising your child with an eye toward who they will be as a 35-year-old.

Some parents approach child-rearing to avoid judgment from community members. Might you have determined you will never become a topic of their judgment?

- Has your fear been stoked that your child will fall behind if they don't participate in every activity? Your job is to build secure children, not to satisfy people who have no idea how you really parent. Reassure yourself that you are parenting for genuine long-term success. Your 35-year-old will be well prepared for the world because they learned to think wisely and independently under your loving guidance. Your child will be prepared for their second job because they are raised to be collaborative and respond well to constructive feedback.

- Have you been made to believe that children are destined for trouble without strict parental oversight? First, remember that children also want to be safe, and they appreciate guidance on how to make wise decisions. Further, rest assured that a Lighthouse Parent offers oversight, including rules, to keep their children safe from true physical or emotional dangers. But keeping your child safe in the long-run includes them learning from real-life consequences within challenging (but still safe) territories. For example, you would never stand passively by if your child were becoming involved with a peer group that heavily used substances. But you would let them participate with peers in school-related activities, even if some of their peer interactions were challenging.

Building Real Confidence

You've tried to find that balance between ensuring safety and allowing for safe exploration from the time your infant was crawling. You trusted then that children learn best when they "stretch" into new territory and can handle something they hadn't imagined they could. But you also noticed that they felt secure taking chances when they saw that you were watching and knew that what they were attempting to do was safe for them. They ventured into new territory but kept checking back to see that you were still monitoring their progress, scanning the environment for dangers. They read your unspoken signals to be sure you still approved and didn't seem worried. Even then, you acted as a lighthouse—a reliable presence that allowed them to learn to trust their newfound abilities.

In any moment, hovering may pull you to the familiar and make you feel better. But draw from the lessons you learned as you've witnessed the miracles of development. Children must do as much on their own as they can handle; that is the way that lessons take hold and the confidence to conquer the next challenge is built.

CHAPTER 15

Steer Them Away From the Rocks, While Watching From a Distance

Why keep a distance rather than hovering nearby? Distance offers you an expansive view. This can empower you with advance warnings to prevent problems before they become crises. Further, your distance itself communicates to your child that you believe they have the capability and self-interest to learn to scan for danger themselves.

Just as you never let your toddler put their hand on the stove or run into the street, you will never allow your child to place themselves at great risk. However, most of your protective actions won't involve grabbing them urgently by the hand or emphatically shouting, "No!" Instead, whenever possible, as a Lighthouse Parent, you will steer them away from the rocks before they come close to crashing against them. Your longer-term goal is for them to be self-protective so they will intuitively steer a wide berth away from the rocks.

Preparing for Adolescence

Adolescents are natural explorers who are wired to stretch into new territories. When our children learn to trust that we only say "no" in cases of true danger, as adolescents, they will better trust our safety-based concerns.

Shaping Your Lifelong Bond

Adults never grow out of appreciating our loved ones for being concerned about us. Our desire to feel protected remains throughout our lives. But adults can resent overprotection or restriction. When your child sees you as protective but not controlling, they will be more likely to see you as someone to turn toward to (re)experience the comfort of human protection.

The Power of the Word "No"

We offer our children a gift when we raise them with as few noes as possible. Yes, to exploring the world. Yes, to stretching into new territories. Yes, to trying on different hats to imagine how to best fit in the world. Using limits judiciously does more than leave room for these critical yeses. Children rely on our limits to define the boundaries within which they *can* safely explore. For that reason, our thoughtfully used "no" enables the stretching that defines healthy development. The carefully balanced use of yeses and noes encourages and protects your child!

Too many parents use the word "no" when they really mean "maybe" or "I'm too tired or busy to consider something now." Consequently, when they need to use that word urgently ("No, you may not get into the car with an unsafe driver!") or to set a nonnegotiable boundary ("No, you may not go to your friend's house without adult supervision!") parents may not be believed. Instead, children raised with half-hearted limits learn to beg, argue, and wear their parents down until they say, "Well, maybe," and finally, "Yes." In these cases, how could we expect children to know when a situation merits a hard and fast "no!"? Critically, children may have learned to rely on their own judgment (before it is trustworthy) because their parents have said no to things of little consequence and later changed their minds anyway.

Your child must understand, "My parent only says 'no' if it really matters, and therefore I must trust them and follow their guidance." To be clear, there is nothing wrong with saying, "Maybe," or "I'll have to think about it." That is a clear signal that the decision will be made later. I would encourage you to welcome your child's input in "maybe" discussions, as this will give them the opportunity to understand what responsibility or safety measures they need to demonstrate to shift you comfortably into the "yes" column.

Saying "no" is a social skill to be learned

Many of us find it uncomfortable to assert ourselves, especially in relationships we care about. How you use the word "no" will make a difference in whether your child comfortably includes it in their communication toolkit. If you use the word apologetically and with some degree of guilt like, "No, I'm sorry," your child may learn to feel badly when they need to make a stand. If you imply you need permission to say no, "I said no! OK?" your child may learn that holding firm is inherently uncomfortable. On the other hand, when you use the word rarely but know that its use communicates genuine caring and commitment to protecting a loved one, your child will recognize and appreciate its value and power.

In Chapter 30, we'll discuss the importance of preparing your child to say "no" as an essential communication tool to navigate pressures while ensuring they adhere to their own standards. For now, remember your children are learning the power of the word from you.

Limits for different situations

In the case of **true danger**, act and explain later. There may be no time for words. If you use words, make them short, clear, and nonnegotiable, like, "No, you may not—this is about safety." If emotions are running high, your child may not be able to process the explanation anyway. There will be time later when safety is assured that you can explain your decision and attend to their emotions.

In **nonemergency situations**, your judicious noes and clear limits fall into several categories.

1. **"No, and this will never change."** Explain why this hard limit is based on safety or values and will never change. Make yourself clear, leaving no room for misunderstanding. An example in this category is the use of illicit substances. "No, it will never be acceptable for you to smoke cigarettes because it seriously damages your health."

2. **"No, you are not yet able to handle this."** The path is clearly set that when your child demonstrates responsibility, they will be able to earn more privileges. An example here might be your child asking to go to the mall without adult supervision. A "no" in this category is best handled by fleshing out the meaning of the word "yet." Be as specific as you can on the steps your child can take to earn this privilege. Refer to Chapters 16 and 28 for strategies on helping young people grasp that they earn privileges when they demonstrate they are ready to handle them.

3. **"No, this puts too much stress on the family right now."** This teaches that what might be desired for the individual might not be possible because the needs of others must be considered. An example of this is not allowing a sleepover in your home while an older sibling is preparing for an exam. While these temporary limits might feel disappointing, they also teach the concept of compromising in recognition of others' needs. This prepares children to lead families of their own and to be good workplace colleagues and productive community members.

In Chapter 16, we will discuss the role of the words "maybe" and "yes!" in encouraging and shaping your child.

Attend to Feelings Without Creating Confusion or Fear

Children need to understand the whys behind our actions to learn to make decisions for themselves. But be careful that your explanations do not create confusion. Explain what value you are upholding, but do not apologize for your decision. Even if they look disappointed, avoid messages like "I'm sorry that I'm not able to allow you to do what you want," because the message can be confusing. You're not sorry, you're doing this to protect them!

Children deserve empathy as they react to our limits. Limits can create disappointment and sadness. This might be especially true if your limits are tighter than those set by your child's friends' parents. You can attend to their feelings without apologizing or entering negotiations. "I know this is hard, but it's my job to keep you safe." Or, "I know you're disappointed, but this is a decision I've made because we need the house to be quiet this weekend."

Focusing on safety and protection ensures that your child understands the reasoning behind your decisions. I want to caution you, however, not to instill fear in your child as you emphasize potential danger. Make the point that we don't need to fear what we've taken the steps to avoid.

Do what your child cannot do: think ahead

The goal is for your child to learn to anticipate problems and steer away from them. That is a skill they will develop when their cognitive (or thinking) development is advanced enough that they can make the leap between present actions and future consequences. For now, your child needs you to predict possible problems and consider which of your child's actions may lead—step by step—to undesired future outcomes.

Your child deserves to learn why you are making decisions today based on something that may occur tomorrow. But their current thinking abilities, assuming they are a preadolescent, may not allow them to easily understand your conclusions. And a lecture that ties together each step and leaps to dire consequences will activate their stress responses but not their thinking capacity. Use the strategy discussed in Chapter 11 to guide your child to understand how and why you are making decisions to steer them away from danger. And remember, even if you have acted out of justified fear, wait until you are calm before you attempt to help your child understand your decision. Otherwise, you will be unable to co-regulate with them. Without you as a calm, steady presence, their emotional brain will dominate, making it difficult for their thinking brain to absorb the lesson.

CHAPTER 16

Everyday Discipline: Always Teaching But Ready With Course Corrections and Corrective Actions

Every day? Wait. You may be viewing discipline as a reaction or punishment in response to something a child does. You may be thinking, "My child doesn't need discipline **every** day!" Discipline should be guiding your approach to parenting—every day—unrelated to any misbehavior. Why? Because the word *discipline* means to teach or guide, and we should regularly be offering our children lessons.

Discipline is about increasing our children's sense of control, not ours. Therefore, we must ensure a child understands the cause-and-effect nature of consequences. If a consequence offers a lesson, because it is tied to their action, it is discipline. If a consequence is out of proportion to their action, it will feel like retribution. If a consequence only makes a child feel badly about what they did, it is a punishment—which is not discipline. A child who feels punished or who concludes their parent is acting not as a guide but out of anger does not learn lessons.

Preparing for Adolescence

When your child learns that demonstrating thoughtful and responsible behaviors earns them more privileges, they will grow to be an adolescent who will seek to stretch their limits while wanting to prove to you they are ready to do so.

118

Shaping Your Lifelong Bond

When you are a source of life lessons delivered in a way that feels affirming rather than controlling, you'll play a role in your child's life for decades to come.

Encouragement

Our children develop by venturing into new territory. With each success and every recovery from failure they gain confidence to stretch further. We should set clear boundaries beyond which they cannot stray but encourage new experiences within those boundaries. In the last chapter, we covered the noes that set the limits. The yeses are just as important to discipline because our encouragement fuels children to explore and grow. We must encourage them to use the gifts of childhood: curiosity, playfulness, and an indefatigable desire to seek new adventures. Our boundaries give them the go-ahead to explore within safe limits, while giving us the comfort to cheer from the sidelines as they do.

The attention a child seeks

Children never stop wanting their parents' attention. They'll usually start by doing the things that delight us, but if that doesn't work, they'll whine or act out. Make sense? Children do what it takes to get the attention they crave. Your child's kindergarten teacher may have told you the secret of parenting the 4- or 5-year-old is to catch them when they're good and redirect them when they're not. I would argue, though, that the most effective disciplinary strategy for a child or adolescent of any age is to notice and reinforce positive behavior.

Shifting your focus

It's easy to grow used to good behaviors and focus our energies on correcting those we don't like. Keep a diary for a few days and note what gets your attention. Do you pay more attention to your child when they are behaving well or when they are not? Once you recognize a pattern, you'll more easily change it.

There is no better way of "teaching" your child than showing appreciation for their positive actions by using *specific* praise. "You're behaving so beautifully today," does not give enough information to underscore what pleases you. Try instead, "I think it was terrific that you helped your little brother with their homework," or, "I noticed how patient you were earlier when I wasn't able to answer your question right away." But positive attention and encouragement isn't the only way to ensure your child learns lessons. They'll also need to learn from their misbehavior. Read on to explore how to discipline when things aren't going well.

Natural consequences

There is no better teacher than life itself. Natural consequences are real-life results that follow our actions. If we leave a mess, we live in a mess. If we don't finish our work, there's less time for play. If we treat someone badly, they'll be less likely to want to spend time with us. If there's not a safety issue or something that could cause enduring emotional harm, allow consequences to play out.

Most of the time, let your child discover the link between their actions and consequences. Occasionally, help them make the connection between their behaviors and outcomes. "I want to take you to the park, but we'll only have time to do that if we take the trash out so it is ready for pickup." Other times you'll reinforce the message after the consequence. "I know you're disappointed that I didn't make it to your game, but I didn't learn about it until this morning. Please give me the schedule earlier so I can show up for you."

Earned privileges

Top-down directives, such as, "You'll do as I say! Why? Because these are the rules!" offer no lessons, just limits. On the other hand, when your child truly practices self-control and gains wise decision-making capacities while stretching into new territories, your disciplinary approach is working. The bottom line is we give children the privileges they can handle while keeping safety nets in place. Once your child learns that privileges are earned, they will do what it takes to demonstrate their worthiness of increased responsibilities, expanded boundaries, and privileges associated with displayed maturity.

Convincing arguments

If your child's limits are based on a rigid set of rules, such as, "You're X-years-old, so this is what you can do," they will not be motivated to demonstrate to you *or prove to themselves* they are ready for more. If your child is a self-advocate (and let's hope that you raised them to be!), they are always going to want a bit more responsibility than they currently have. To get there, they'll push back against your current boundaries hoping you'll expand them. My advice is to let them win these negotiating sessions when they make a reasonable case. Why? In the process of negotiating (OK, occasionally arguing 😊) with you, they'll make the precise case of what they will do to prove they *really* are deserving of the new privilege. "I can _____ because I've shown I can _____." Or, "I am willing to _____, but that should mean I can _____." This kind of communication has 2 clear benefits: 1) They are tying privileges to demonstrated responsibility, essentially setting rules for themselves, and 2) They are learning useful give-and-take skills for future interactions with peers, partners, teachers, colleagues, even bosses.

One more critical point: If your rules are rigid and your child learns that their positive actions earn no reward and convincing arguments are ignored, they may seek out a way to work around the rules.

Mutual Agreements

You might consider holding a family meeting in which your child can state their desired privileges and you (and other caregivers) can clarify your expectations for your child earning *and maintaining* the privilege. You can also set expectations of how your child should contribute to household functioning. Many families record these discussions in written agreements. Written agreements have 2 advantages. First, their formality can motivate a child to thoroughly consider their commitments. Second, when people inevitably have different memories of the same discussion, a written record can prevent many arguments.

These discussions are opportune moments to distinguish those "No, and this will never change" rules from the "No, you are not able to handle this *yet*" rules as discussed in Chapter 15. Your child should know that a permanent "no" is because that situation is *never* safe, while most restrictions will be loosened as they demonstrate their capabilities to wisely manage increasing independence. Your goal is to have the "not yet" category shrink as your child matures.

Ideally, agreements will be revised on a regular basis, perhaps every 2 or 3 months. This allows for a check-in on behavior and newly earned privileges to be added. It also allows you to add new responsibilities for your child to contribute to your household, as they mature. Framed correctly, your child will see their increasing contributions (ie, more sophisticated chores) as demonstrations of your increasing trust. Their contributions will also be frequent reminders of how much they matter (see Chapter 24).

Grasping cause and effect

Sitting down together to think through what your child can handle offers an opportunity to have them assess their own competencies. For example, your child might make a request while explaining, "I think I can handle this because I am good at doing _____." Further, because they'll earn increasing privileges only if they successfully handle current ones, guide them to ask for only what they believe they can master. This process prepares them for the one-step-at-a-time framework to their growing independence, as we will discuss in Chapter 28. Finally, they may consider what ongoing supports they need before confidently and safely venturing forth. Together, this all helps your child develop cause-and-effect thinking. They'll understand that their actions are linked to a favorable or unfavorable outcome; they earn their privilege or demonstrate they are not yet ready for it.

The following is a sample of what an agreement might look like. Liam is a responsible 11-year-old who takes his schoolwork seriously and is a loving (usually) sibling to his 2 younger sisters. As you review, do not focus on Liam's requests, because your child's requests will differ based on their age, desires, and the community in which you live. Instead, focus on the back-and-forth nature of the agreements and the opportunity to understand a child's wishes and tie them to parents' desires to see them stay safe and demonstrate responsibility.

Notice these agreements are a means to deliver lessons because the child understands the whys behind the decisions. Drive the lessons home by allowing your child to run through what-if scenarios. "What if I come home after curfew and haven't called?" "What if I am late but called to tell you how I was managing a problem?" This process helps clarify the purpose of the rules and allows your child to understand that you'll be most flexible when made aware of changing circumstances.

Liam's Agreement to Earn Privileges

Liam's Request for New Privileges	Parent(s) Response
I'd like to be able to stay over at Scott's house while his parents travel on the weekends.	No. We will never let you stay in a home without adult supervision. That is not safe.
I'd like to be able to ride my bike to the mall with my friends.	You are not yet ready for this privilege. It involves crossing some streets with heavy and unpredictable traffic and it will be dark by the time you come home. You'll be able to do this when you are a bit older. You are ready now to go to the mall by yourself with friends, and we are happy to make sure you get a ride back and forth.
I'd like to extend my curfew from 7:15 pm until 8:00 pm. (Example discussion: "I've shown that I'm getting my homework and chores done. I'd like more time with my friends.)	We think you can handle this, but we'll need to be sure that • We know where you are. • You'll call or text us if you'll be late. • You'll use our code word to contact one of us if you are in an uncomfortable situation and need our support (see Chapter 30). • You'll need to complete your homework. This means if you have a lot of homework, you'll need to finish it before you go out or return home earlier. (Example discussion: "You'll lose this privilege if the quality of your homework slips.") • You still complete your household chores.
I'd like to not have a required bedtime anymore.	We agree you can handle more flexibility, but you need quality sleep to function in school. We can't agree to no bedtime requirement but can agree to mandatory lights out no later than 10:30 pm. You stay alert in school and focused in extracurricular activities to demonstrate you're getting enough sleep. Your cell phone and computer remain docked in the charging station.
Parent(s) Request for Liam to Increase Contributions	**Liam's Response**
We need you to mow the lawn and rake the leaves. This takes pressure off us and saves the household money.	No problem. I appreciate my allowance and know that this is how I earn it. I also feel good about saving you money. (Example discussion: "Is there anything else I can do to earn extra money for the game console I'm saving up for?")
We need you to walk your sister from the bus to her first classroom every morning. This helps us know she will get there safely.	I will always do that. I like keeping her safe. She's sometimes a pain at home, but she always makes me feel like she's proud of me as a big brother at school.
Signed	Date

Consequences *should* make sense

You want your child to feel consequences are reasonable and fair responses to their behavior. When they can look at an agreement and see that they have not held up their end of the bargain, it will make sense that they cannot maintain the privilege. This will be discussed in the part of this chapter where we cover corrective actions. For now, understand that a mutual agreement in which your child grasps the connection between their behavior and their privileges creates a road map for when your child is not meeting expectations. For example, suppose Liam doesn't dock his electronic devices in the charging station and is found to be gaming at midnight. He has lost the privilege of having less supervision around bedtime. He would need to return to lights out at 10:00 pm when you are awake to supervise him putting away his electronics.

Who's got the power?

Partnering with your child doesn't give your authority away. A child engaged in self-advocacy will keep communication open and their parents will likely know more about their life. Further, the more input your child has in thinking about what actions demonstrate responsibility, the more likely they will understand appropriate consequences. Above all, your child will be motivated to meet your expectations and even impress you with how much they can handle. See? This approach actually increases your influence.

Course corrections

Course corrections are supportive actions you take *before* a problem occurs in the hope that you can steer your child in a better direction. When you are worried, explore the whys behind your child's concerning behavior. Remember, depending on your child's developmental stage, they may not be able to grasp or explain the whys driving their actions. Use a series of questions that explore what they are feeling or experiencing when they behave in a certain manner (see Chapter 11, the part titled "Getting to Why and How"). The course correction will differ depending on what is driving your child's behaviors.

If your child's changing behavior is related to stress, anxiety, or sadness, seek professional support early. A child-serving professional can help them build strategies to manage uncomfortable or distressing thoughts or feelings (see Chapter 22).

If your child cannot foresee the consequences of their actions, you have 2 options depending on the circumstances.

1. Trust natural consequences to teach the lesson, and as consequences begin playing out, underscore them with discussions to make sure your child absorbs the cause-and-effect nature of the consequences.
2. Help them understand the consequences of their actions by playing them out in a conversation they can understand. Avoid the lecture; instead, use strategies discussed in Chapter 11 in the part titled "Working Toward That 'Aha!'"

If you believe peers are having a negative influence on your child, respond before their influence deepens. If it is a mild problem, equipping your child with peer negotiation skills may suffice (see Chapters 29 and 30). If the peer group is dangerous or emotionally destructive, take a more aggressive stand. It is difficult to demand they never see their problematic peers again, so immediate separation must be reserved for extreme circumstances. But you can always facilitate a shift in peer influence by helping your child find a new set of friends. Ensure exposure to children in multiple settings (for example, school, playing fields, after-school activities, religious and cultural groups, extended family). Having multiple circles of friends should begin early but becomes deeply protective in middle school when peers take on greater influence and friend groups change rapidly, often causing a great deal of distress. If one group drifts away, your child will not be left isolated if they have already fostered connections with another group.

Corrective Actions

Corrective actions are the consequences we give in response to a misbehavior or demonstration of irresponsibility. Consequences must be delivered alongside the message, "You've done something wrong, and I reject that behavior, but I love you." When we reinforce our love is unconditional, even as we clearly state when we find a behavior unacceptable, our children will know it is safe to turn to us when they find themselves in trouble.

Parents who are responsive to what their child can manage will use discipline most effectively. Rigid rules don't allow for growth, and rigid punishments not directly tied to what the child has done don't teach lessons. You can expand boundaries and offer more privileges as your child successfully demonstrates growth. In other words, the best corrective actions are not those that make your child feel your anger or suffer from their mistakes but are those that return their privileges to the point that they were able to handle them.

Corrective actions should teach a lesson and do so best through a consequence that reinforces personal accountability. In a child's mind, when a corrective action feels worse than the "crime," they'll focus on how "unfair" they are being treated, which will prevent them from seeing their role in earning the consequence. Instead, they receive the message, "You aren't in control. We, your parents, control you." This flies in the face of a major goal of development—to have our child gain a sense of control over their destiny.

Cell phone access used as a corrective action

Cell phones are often a parent's go-to consequence because they are easily restricted or taken away, without causing real harm. However, taking away a cell phone or screentime is no longer a minor consequence to young people. It is their social lifeline and is often used for homework. Therefore, limiting or restricting electronic devices makes sense when the misbehavior is logically tied to cell phone or screentime use. Even then, however, you may need to come up with a plan that recognizes the necessity of internet access for homework or the phone for emergency communication.

The loss of electronic devices will be seen as a punishment if the misbehavior or display of irresponsibility was unrelated to a phone or screen. For example, Shelly was supposed to come home right after school because her father needed help around the house to prepare for her birthday party the next day. She excitedly talked to her friends about it after school and completely lost track of time. Instead, she came home later than she agreed to. When her father took away her phone for 3 days, she stormed out of the room in anger. Although she still hosts her party the next day, she does so while feeling saddened because she didn't get to talk about it with her friends the night before and is angry that her father ruined the party. As mentioned, Shelly sees this more as a punishment instead of a lesson.

The loss of cell phone privileges will offer a lesson if the problem behavior is related to electronic devices. For example, Jonah recently began staying up late gaming with people across the world. He knew that he couldn't get on the computer until his homework was completed; thus, he consistently finished his work before going on. Soon, Jonah made a friend across the world and began gaming with him after school (12 time zones away). Jonah was gaming between 3:00 and 6:00 am every morning. His grades started to slip, and he fell asleep in school. His parents took away his electronic access for 2 weeks except for homework use. Later, they returned his phone and computer but insisted both be docked in the living room charger at 10:00 pm. At first, Jonah was upset because he missed gaming. But then he noticed that he was doing better in school and appreciated his parents for noticing and responding to his mistake.

Grounding used correctly and incorrectly as a corrective action

Grounding a child may offer a sense of relief to parents who are frightened by a child's behavior because at least for a while they don't have to worry about their child's whereabouts. But to a child, it is a very big deal because it restricts them entirely from their social lives and interferes with their inborne developmental need to stretch their wings.

Grounding will be seen as a punishment if the misbehavior or display of irresponsibility is unrelated to the fact that the child was not at home being closely watched. For example, Deion was supposed to come home after school but didn't arrive until 6:30 pm. He was trying out for the school play but didn't want to tell his parents until he got the part. He didn't respond to texts because he was reading scripts and left his silenced phone in his jacket. His parents were distraught because he usually always responds to their check-ins. They were activating the community watch group when he walked in unaware of their concern. Relieved, they shouted, "Deion, you're grounded for a week!" To his parents, grounding their son made sense because they were imagining tremendous peril and anything that protected him from danger seemed wise. Deion had a different experience. He knew he was never in danger and was, in fact, doing something positive. The punishment made no sense to him. He left the room angry, deciding not to tell his parents that he just got an important role in the play, and decides he'll sneak out of the house.

Grounding will offer a lesson if your child put themselves at risk because they were away from adult supervision. It ensures the child will be closely watched and kept away from a worrisome behavior. For example, Lizette's behavior had been changing. Now a sixth grader, her best friend since kindergarten was Sadie. Recently, both girls had tried to join a new set of friends. Lizette started dressing differently, returned home later than expected, and snuck into her room. She was sometimes disrespectful and shut down conversations easily. Sadie's mother called Lizette's mother and shared that her daughter behaved similarly and that she discovered marijuana Sadie had hidden under her bed. The parents agreed they needed to sort out where this influence—and drugs—were coming from. The girls were grounded while their parents took actions to ensure safety. They framed the restrictions in the language of caring and protection. Lizette expressed how angry she was and that she resented that she wasn't trusted. But she went into her room and cried out of relief. Now she could tell this new set of "friends" that she was grounded and being watched closely. She told them she was not able to smoke again.

Framework for corrective actions and incentives for growth

Agreements that create a road map for earning privileges will not prevent all problems but can anticipate many of them. Because agreements essentially say, "I'll earn this privilege by being responsible and will maintain it by continually demonstrating my responsibility," children understand they will lose their privileges when they don't display responsibility. You've clarified precisely what conditions you need met to be comfortable with them stretching into new territory. This simplifies arriving at consequences. If your child doesn't follow the plan, you revoke the privilege until they demonstrate responsibility long enough to earn it back.

As previously mentioned, return a privilege to the point your child mastered in the past. This works seamlessly for privileges related to time. For example, if Liam doesn't notify his parents when he'll be later than expected, he'll lose the privilege of the 8:00 pm curfew. He would return to the point where he demonstrated responsibility, a 7:15 pm curfew. This approach helps children understand that they, not you, determine whether their privileges expand. You are letting them operate at the limits of their demonstrated responsibility. We want our children to see themselves as decision-makers and problem-solvers who largely control their destiny!

When you revisit the agreement every 2 or 3 months, you create an incentive system. Your child will know what they must do to continue to stretch to their limits. They'll do what it takes to ensure that they adhere to the agreements in the hope that next time their privileges will expand further. Bonus: They also may learn the vital life lesson that delaying immediate gratification often leads to attaining a longer-term goal.

Rules Children and Teens Can Live By

Your child may resist your rules or resent your expectations if they are stricter than those of other parents in your child's circle of friends. So don't do this alone! Talk to other parents and hold your children to high and fair expectations. If you set common expectations, your child will more likely see them as "what other kids do too." They can meet your expectations, stay safe, and feel "normal" at the same time.

CHAPTER 17

Anticipating the Opportunity Adolescence Offers

Many parents of school-aged children or early tweens worry about adolescence approaching. They may fear the loss of childhood. They may imagine that their child who looks up to them will grow to resent them. They may worry about risk and fear their child making a mistake that will take a heavy toll. These fears are created in us by a culture that negatively stereotypes adolescents. These concerns are stoked by others who tell us to "hang on tight." They are solidified by experts who focus on the problems without telling you how special the adolescent years can be for parents and who fail to tell you that you will remain the most important and trusted guide in your tween or teen's life.

What thoughts come to your mind when *you* think of teens? How we think of adolescents affects our attitude about them and our actions toward them. That's why when you hear "teen" or "adolescent," I want you to think, "What an opportunity that awaits!"

When you see adolescence as an "opportunity," you'll be reminded that your child is full of **potential.** Recognizing their potential, when your child becomes an adolescent, you'll wisely seek advice from the expert who knows the most about your child: your adolescent. And when you want to learn more, you'll steer clear of "experts" who will suggest adolescence is a time to survive. You'll reject this view because you want to make the most of this opportunity, not make your way through it while holding your breath.

Preparing for Adolescence

Your child absorbs your every emotion and their ability to do so will intensify as adolescence approaches. If you fear the loss of childhood, so will they. If you expect a diminished relationship, so will they. Instead, look forward to a growing—albeit changing—relationship and your teen will more likely grow into that stronger relationship with you.

Shaping Your Lifelong Bond

Your unconditional and unwavering parental presence remains the bedrock of your lifelong bond. The adolescent years are a time of change when children need the stability of a loving parent as much or more than ever. Young people need to distance themselves a bit from parents as they learn to trust they could stand on their own, if they wanted to. But when parents withdraw from them, precisely when they are most needed, it is deeply confusing. If you remain emotionally present while also honoring increasing independence, your child will always remember you stood by them and want you to continue to do so throughout your lives.

Think Productively

"Opportunity" may not *yet* be the way you frame adolescence. But investing in seeing adolescence in a positive light is critical to ensuring that you remain an irreplaceable guide in your child's life. Adolescents have a remarkable sensitivity to what others are feeling even when words remain unspoken and actions are controlled. I assure you that your teen's desire to please you will remain strong. If your teen senses that your view of them changes, it could affect the expectations they set for themself. Their internal voice might say, "Well, if teens are supposed to be (fill in the blank), then I'll be that way too."

When you think of adolescence, use productive thoughts (left column of table on page 131) to replace stereotyped thoughts (right column). This may be most important during challenging moments. I never want you to fall into the trap of explaining unacceptable behavior as "teens being teens." Instead, understand those behaviors in a larger context that often reflects the pain or confusion in your child's life. With this approach, your relationship can grow stronger through the toughest times. Adolescence is not a time to get past, but actually is a time when your involvement makes all the difference. Your teen needs you to continue to believe the best of them!

Productive thoughts![a]	Undermining thoughts about adolescence . . .
A time when adults are carefully observed and serve as role models	A time when adults are rejected
A time when teens are learning to relate to people outside the family	A time when teens only care about friends
An opportunity to grow and develop	A period teens must survive
An opportunity for parents to engage with and shape their teens	A time parents must survive
A period when sensitivity is developing and empathy is growing	A time of high and unpredictable emotions
A time of remarkable development	A time of so many changes
A time to learn from challenges	A painful time
A time of working to gain increased independence	A time of rebellion
A time for teens to test and expand limits and for adults to set protective boundaries	A risky time
A time to gain lessons and earn wisdom	A time to get past

[a] Note that the productive thoughts about teens are developed fully in *Congrats—You're Having a Teen! Strengthen Your Family and Raise a Good Person.*

Telling the truth about teens

Our culture tells an inaccurate story about teens that creates lowered expectations for them. In fact, Christy Buchanan, PhD, of Wake Forest University, has shown that parents' lowered expectations of teens predict worse parent-child relationships, more risk-taking, and challenging behaviors over time. In other words, our attitudes shape the way we interact with our children and therefore the way they end up behaving.

Let's call out these inaccurate descriptions of adolescents—myths—and replace them with the truths. Myths hurt teens because they grow in a world that sees them through a distorted lens. But will these myths really harm your teen or your relationship? Yes! Because if you believe them, you may conclude that what you do doesn't matter. After all, if your teen doesn't care what you think, why stay involved? If you view teens as people who can't be reasoned with, why would you bother guiding them to think things through? If you believe that your teen is destined to be risky, why not focus your energy on placing restrictions on them in a desperate attempt to protect them? But tight restrictions placed out of fear will deny your child the ability to grow, to stretch, and to sometimes learn from mistakes under your watchful eyes.

The truth about teens[a]	The myths to reject
Adults are the most important people in the lives of young people, and teens like adults. In fact, adolescents care more about what their parents think than they care about anybody else's opinion.	Adolescents don't care what adults think and dislike their parents.
Adolescence is a time of astoundingly rapid brain development, and we can shape our children's future far into adulthood by nurturing that development.	By adolescence, a young person's development is on autopilot.
Adolescents are super learners, and they will learn more during this period of their life than at any other time that follows.	Adolescents are lazy and don't care much about what they learn. They'd rather hang out with friends and have fun.
As super learners, adolescents are driven to explore limits and to peek beyond the edges to gain new knowledge. Because danger may exist beyond those edges, adult guidance is needed. Young people care about safety and want to avoid danger and therefore welcome adult guidance when it is clearly meant to keep them safe.	Adolescents think they are invincible and are wired for risk.
Teens can be as rational and thoughtful as adults. To take advantage of this capability, we need to talk to them calmly, in a manner that acknowledges their intelligence and recognizes that they are the experts in their own lives.	Adolescents are driven by emotion, and it is hard to talk sense into them.
Adolescents are driven by idealism and committed to repairing the world. They find meaning and purpose when given the opportunity to serve.	Adolescents are self-centered and selfish.
Parents matter as much to their teen's healthy development as when their children were toddlers. They make the most difference through their unconditional presence and wise guidance.	Teens prefer to figure things out on their own. Because they are inherently rebellious, they are uninterested in what their parents think, say, or do.

[a] Note that the truths about teens are developed fully in *Congrats—You're Having a Teen! Strengthen Your Family and Raise a Good Person.*

More to Love

Your children are growing. They couldn't stop developing even if they wanted to. If your older children and tweens sense that you are anticipating their next step of development with dread, they'll fear or resent their own growth. Let them know that you look forward to seeing the young adult that is taking shape and always appreciate their growth—inside and out—because it gives you more of them to love.

You'll Be Well Prepared

You'll be well prepared for adolescence. One of the key reasons you're becoming a Lighthouse Parent is to put into place those strategies that will make adolescence smoother for you and your child. As your child approaches the teen years, read my book, *Congrats—You're Having a Teen! Strengthen Your Family and Raise a Good Person,* for the next steps in applying your parenting skills. It features lots of strategies to make the most out of the opportunity the teen years offer.

One more key point is that adolescence is a time where development is moving a mile a minute. Bodies are changing. Emotions are rising to the surface. Core issues of identity are materializing. This undoubtedly is a time to take an active role in shaping the adult coming into focus. A Lighthouse Parent is a stable force on the shoreline. When you serve as stability during a time filled with so many changes, you will forever be seen as someone worth counting on for your reliable presence. As a result, perhaps above all, adolescence is an opportunity to strengthen your relationship for a lifetime.

Part 5

Resilience and Thriving

I choose to be a Lighthouse Parent . . . I'll look into the waves and trust they'll learn to ride them.

CHAPTER 18

Human Connection: The Core Ingredient of Resilience and Thriving

Dr Veronica Svetaz and Dr Tamera Coyne-Beasley join me in writing this chapter on human connection. They are 2 of the visionaries in adolescent medicine, both have parented children of Color and both are personal heroes of mine. No chapter on the power of our interconnections could make sense if not written by people who bring the strength of diverse cultures together.

Resilience is the capacity to adapt from challenges and gain strength in the process. It has been described as "ordinary magic."[1] The human capability to adapt is, indeed, magical. And the fact that we possess this innate ability does make it ordinary. But the magic does not appear from nowhere. It is rooted in the power of human beings to support others through challenges and to instill within them the understanding that we all ultimately belong to one another.

Resilience may strengthen us, but *maintaining* resilience through difficult situations can be exhausting. Our goal is not to be resilient—to be able to bounce back—it must be to **THRIVE**. When human connection is what contributes to our resilience, we are strengthened because we are enriched by those relationships. We learn that others care about us while realizing our presence enhances

---

1. Masten A. *Ordinary Magic: Resilience in Development.* The Guilford Press; 2015.

their lives. It may tire us to remain resilient, but when we stand with others, we secure the relationships that are key to human thriving.

Preparing for Adolescence

Identity development involves answering the question, "Who am I?" This is one of the main tasks of adolescence. When an adolescent knows that they are part of a family, community, and culture, they feel connected, and part of that daunting question is answered.

Shaping Your Lifelong Bond

If you raise your child to feel connected to people and to have healthy pride in your culture, being a member of your family will be a central part of their identity. If they choose to have children, they will want to pass along those connections. Regardless of whether they have children, you will become someone who shares family history and wisdom.

Why Connection Matters

Too many people have been told that strong people can go at it alone. Often people who were raised in dysfunctional families or have been mistreated in relationships have learned that self-reliance is a necessity. Then, in a well-earned effort to ensure their own children don't let people take advantage of them, they raise them to believe that they should never be reliant on anyone but themselves.

It is possible that you are one of those children raised to see self-reliance as a virtuous display of inner strength. Now, you have a child of your own and may want to pass along that wisdom. If any of the circumstances in the previous paragraph describe you, I am suggesting you pause and reflect. *Do not pass along the resilience lessons born from pain.*

I, too, want your child to be strong. I want them to have the strength to surmount challenges and to have such high self-esteem that they would *never* let someone mistreat them. That kind of strength comes from knowing you are deserving of respect. When we are open with our children about our love for them, it instills within them the understanding that they are worthy of being loved. This positions them for healthy relationships throughout their life and will shield them from toxic ones.

Being able to be independent and self-reliant at times is undoubtedly a strength. *Choosing* mutual interdependence with others at times is key both to human survival and thriving.

People need to know they belong

The journey from childhood through adolescence and into adulthood is about forming a sense of identity, an understanding of who you are, and how you fit in. Simply, it is about answering the most fundamental of human questions: "Who am I?" This question has many subparts, including

- How do I fit in with my peers?
- How will I support my family?
- How will I contribute to my community?
- Who am I as a member of my culture? Faith? Community?
- How have I been shaped by my ancestors who have preceded me, and how do I leave something meaningful for my descendants?

When we stand beside our children through difficult moments and celebrate with them in triumphant ones, they learn that they are not on this journey alone. It tells them they belong. It reinforces that relationships strengthen us. Being the root of this kind of security and the source of this deep-seated protection ensures your relationship will continue to strengthen long after your child has left your home.

The Resilience Lesson We Teach

When we join with others, we gain strength and simultaneously lend strength to others. To adapt Aesop's "The Bundle of Sticks" fable: A child was feeling frightened and powerless, close to her breaking point. Sometimes this showed through her words, sometimes through tears, and often through silence. A caring adult approached and lovingly explained, "We all get scared sometimes and it may even feel as though we have little control over our lives. Sometimes it even feels as though we might snap like a frail stick." The adult then asks her to pick up a stick lying on the ground. She easily breaks it in 2, relating to its fragility. The adult gathers several sticks, binds them together, and offers them to the child. "Try to break this bundle of sticks." She can barely get them to bend. The adult gently explains, "Each stick by itself can easily break, but when joined with others, they become stronger than their individual strengths. We are like this bundle of sticks. Each of us can be fragile at any moment but joined together we grow stronger. When we feel most vulnerable, we gather people around us to draw from their strengths. Sometimes you will borrow others' strength and often you'll lend your strength to them."

We *are* more powerful together than the sum of our individual strengths. When times get tough, we unify. We hold those we love near and offer those who are vulnerable the extra support they deserve.

Can Loneliness Really Harm Us?

Simply put, yes. In fact, loneliness was highlighted in a surgeon general's report[2] as harming our emotional and physical health. It was not surprising that the report highlighted the association between loneliness and depression, anxiety, and addiction. Its astounding findings also included the fact that loneliness was associated with a greater risk of heart disease, dementia, stroke, and premature death. The impact on lifespan of being socially disconnected was similar to smoking 15 cigarettes daily! It concludes with an inspirational and true statement: "Our individual relationships are an untapped resource—a source of healing hiding in plain sight."

What if my child (or I) like solitude?

People have different temperaments. Some of us are introverted, needing our own space to recharge while others draw energy from others. It is not wrong to be quiet or to need alone time to reflect, think, and recharge. You cannot force human connection on others. However, we all do benefit from trusted, secure

2. *Our Epidemic of Loneliness and Isolation: The US Surgeon General's Advisory on the Healing Effects of Social Connection and Community.* 2023. https://www.hhs.gov/surgeongeneral/priorities/connection/index.html. Accessed August 29, 2024.

relationships. Not everyone needs to be surrounded by a crowd, but everyone deserves deep, trusting relationships.

Do not force human connection but be sure your child is not self-isolating for fear of rejection. Some children are slow starters. They may avoid making friends or opening up on our desired timeline. But with time, they will tentatively try to make friends and find others with whom they can connect. If your child seems more comfortable on the periphery of family gatherings, let them know their presence is welcomed.

Even for the child who prefers quiet, be their lighthouse—that stable force on the shoreline they can always find. When you show them through your unwavering supportive presence that people strengthen one another, they'll eventually learn to reach out to others.

Strength from our community and wisdom from our cultures

A lighthouse sits atop a firm foundation ensuring it will not be washed away from stormy seas. That foundation is laid on rich soil containing deep roots. These roots are your connection to those who surround you in your communities and your cultural heritage inherited from your ancestors. None of us must walk this journey alone; we can draw strength from our communities and wisdom from our cultures.

One of the most critical protective factors for a human being, particularly for one still growing up, is a clear sense of identity. This helps them understand who they are and how to present themselves to the world. Cultural and community identity is a key part of this developing sense of self. Parents can infuse a healthy sense of cultural identity into their children by celebrating their roots, experiencing their rituals and customs, and understanding why certain things are done differently in their community.

As a parent, you are fueled by the pride and knowledge of who your ancestors were, the stories that made your family be, and how the elders transmitted love to you. When you awaken your realization that you are an ancestor too, that you are the main vessel filling your children with that pride, it's a reminder that you are raising your child to be part of something bigger. Our goal is to raise our children to feel connected with their own identity and take pride in their roots so they can stand tall, loving each of the reasons they are unique, not only as an individual but as a member of their culture.

Sometimes elements of our society undermine our sense of worth and rather than appreciate how our diversity strengthens the broader community and nation, society chooses to treat people from different cultures as "the other"—people who do not belong. Your job as a parent is to help buffer your child from these undermining messages. It takes time and concerted investment, but it starts with being intentional about finding people from similar cultures and joining forces in celebrating your history and your strengths. Together you encourage your children to claim their pride, to claim their right to dream, and to dream big as an act of great courage. These acts of courage, collectively, are what move us closer to a just, equitable, and caring society. We offer a deep dive into strategies to build resilient children in the face of racism and other undermining forces in *Building Resilience in Children and Teens: Giving Kids Roots and Wings* in Chapter 22, "Raising Youth of Color in a Complex World."

While we highlight the imperative of each of us finding healthy pride within our cultures, part of our duty is also to pass on a genuine respect toward others and support of others learning about their culture. Just as we support our children to learn about our own histories, we should foster within them a healthy curiosity to learn about the cultures in other communities. This builds on their idealism and their respect for others will help them see themselves as cocreators of a better world.

*   *   *   *   *   *

As each child asks, "Do I belong?" the answer must be a resounding "Yes!" We must raise our children to know that they are connected—that they belong—in so many ways and on so many levels, to our families, to our cultures, and to our communities. Above all, we must raise our children to know that we are all interconnected to each other.

CHAPTER 19

Resilience 101: Foundations of Resilience

It is the security a Lighthouse Parent provides that is the root of a child's resilience. Central to that security is your trust in their ability to ultimately learn to navigate choppy, if not turbulent, waters. Raising children to be resilient in the face of challenges has great value, but our goal is to raise children *prepared to thrive*. To that end, we must hold the vision of building a society that poses fewer challenges to our children's healthy development. The goal is to build a society where every person can reach their potential.

Preparing for Adolescence

Adolescence is a time of many changes when our children doubt themselves. The root of their resilience is to know that our love is unconditional. It is also a time of great potential stress, and we want our children to turn to healthy ways to manage that stress rather than to dangerous quick fixes.

Shaping Your Lifelong Bond

Every human needs resilience-building strategies in their life. Your child will benefit both by your teaching these skills to them and modeling how they help you manage your life. Your adult child will remember you as the person they saw modeling how to work on their own resilience and will turn to you for guidance when they need a resilience boost.

Roots of Resilience

Unconditional love offers deep-seated security that allows children to overcome their own uncomfortable thoughts and feelings and to resist external pressures or undermining messages. It conveys that the person who knows them the most adores them exactly the way they are. It must be repeated often: *Your love says they are worthy of being loved.* Other moments in their life might be unpredictable or painful, but they must know they can never lose you. Unconditional love means that while you won't like all your child's behaviors, you will show up and be supportive during tough times rather than reject them because of a mistaken choice.

Your unwavering love and guaranteed presence offer the security to form deep-trusting future relationships and to launch them into adulthood ready to deal with what may come. It will offer them the self-confidence to stretch into new territory, accept temporary setbacks, and adapt to changing circumstances.

Young people respond to the **expectations** adults set for them. This means we must hold them to high standards. This is about expecting them to be a good human being—their best self. One of the most protective things in a child's life is to be truly known in their best light. When the world pulls your child in the wrong direction, it is your knowledge of who they *really* are that guides them back. As they grow, they will continue to seek your approval while they strengthen and solidify their values. The idea of high expectations can backfire if it is misinterpreted as demanding perfect grades, scores, or trophies. Instead, our expectations about achievements should focus on effort and progress.

You best teach resilience when you **model** how to respond to stress with a wide range of positive coping strategies. We can teach either positive or negative strategies. When we choose harmful ways of managing stress, such as turning to alcohol to relax, our children may follow our example by learning that altering their mood is more efficient than choosing healthier options such as exercise or reaching out to others. When we take healthy steps to calm ourselves, manage life's curveballs, and move forward, they learn people can adapt to tough times. Remember this: You are being constantly watched, and your actions will likely be followed more closely than what you say.

Trust gives our children the safe space to develop their thoughts and test their limits. Children naturally turn to adults for comfort in tough times and we never want that instinct to diminish. However, we also want them to learn to self-comfort and self-regulate. Our trust that they can figure things out and settle themselves is the first step of them gaining the confidence to know they can make wise decisions and learn to trust themselves to adapt. This is why sometimes the best thing we can do is get out of their way, offering our supportive presence and gentle guidance but not the solutions.

Young people need confidence, **belief in oneself**, to take positive steps and to stretch into new territory. They gain that confidence when they feel trusted and have learned they are competent. This is a vital stepping stone to develop the strength to overcome tough times, because they believe they can control what happens to them.

If you wish to consider how to frame all parental interactions in the context of building resilience, read *Building Resilience in Children and Teens: Giving Kids Roots and Wings*.

Seven Critical Cs of Resilience and Positive Development

There are 7 critical Cs—*competence, confidence, connection, character, contribution, coping*, and *control*—that interact to build resilience. I first was inspired to explore these Cs from thought leaders on positive youth development and resilience. The original 4 Cs—*competence, confidence, connection*, and *character*—were proposed by Rick Little, who founded the International Youth Foundation. My perspective has been most influenced by Richard Lerner, PhD, whose research demonstrates that young people who possess these Cs are better poised to thrive. You'll notice the 7 Cs are interrelated and deeply influence one another.

Competence

Competence is about possessing the skill sets that allow people to trust their own judgments, make wise and thoughtful choices, and face challenges. Competencies are not inborn; they are developed and shaped by adults who notice and build on children's existing strengths and teach and model how to gain new skills.

Confidence

Confidence is rooted in competence. As children develop the skill sets that enable them to stretch successfully into new territory, they become, deservedly so, more confident. Confidence cannot be built through false praise; it's something that needs to feel earned. As we notice and underscore their existing strengths, we help them understand they're worthy of increasing confidence.

Connection

Those who are connected to others are more likely to feel a solid sense of security. This produces strong values, enables them to reach to others in difficult times, and may prevent them from seeking undermining relationships. Family is key to security, but connections to people they meet in community, educational, faith, artistic, and athletic settings all contribute to a sense of belonging. Peer relationships are also critical because children thrive with healthy and supportive friendships.

Connection is such a cornerstone of resilience that Chapter 18 is devoted entirely to its value. In truth, Lighthouse Parenting in its entirety is about forming the kind of connection that positions you as an effective guide now and strengthens your family's relationships far into the future.

Character

Character is about having a fundamental sense of right and wrong and a desire to contribute positively to the world. Children and adolescents with character strengths have a strong sense of self-worth and belonging. The feedback they receive when they demonstrate caring toward others underscores how much they matter. Character strengths are essential to thriving and are covered in Chapters 23 through 27.

Contribution

Children who make a difference in others' lives or in their communities receive reinforcing gratitude and are inclined to want to continue earning that gratitude. They may feel more comfortable when they need to receive support because they'll know the giver does not pity or look down on them but gives because they are driven to do so.

Coping

Life can be hard, and we all try to find ways to make it feel easier. But some of the easiest ways to feel better do us harm instead. The best protection, therefore, against turning to unsafe behaviors when under stress is possessing a wide range of positive, adaptive coping strategies to handle life's crises.

Control

The journey toward adulthood is about gaining increasing independence—control over our lives. When children learn their actions lead to real-life consequences, they grow to better consider their choices and, over time, gain impulse control and ultimately true self-control. If parents make all decisions, children are denied opportunities to gain control. A parent's job is to create safe spaces within which children can safely learn self-control while actively giving feedback along the way (see Chapters 15 and 16).

Managing Life's Inevitable Stressors

We relieve discomfort from stress by drawing from familiar coping strategies. Both positive and negative coping strategies work to make us feel better in the short run. Negative strategies work but intensify stress by creating harmful consequences. Despite knowing their harm, many people turn to them because they are quick and easy fixes. But it is precisely because of how instantly and easily they offer relief that many can be addictive. For our children to avoid the dangers posed by these negative quick fixes, they should possess positive coping strategies that *also* reduce discomfort.

Telling children what not to do doesn't work. It denies them the opportunity to share why they are feeling overwhelmed or seeking an escape. Instead, guide them to build healthy strategies while you co-regulate with them to increase their windows of tolerable stress. If your child is already turning to negative coping strategies, stand by them as they learn healthy ways to manage their feelings. If you're reading this when your child is without a worry in the world, *now* is the time to build positive coping skills. This does more than prevent problems; it prepares your child to thrive.

Stress management and coping: taking control when life is challenging

While this plan is about supporting your child to manage stress, much of it will apply to you. This will give you an opportunity to both guide your child and model for them.

There will be times that will demand our full attention and should activate our fight-or-flight responses. Resilient people can focus their concentration and resources on real problems rather than those that are heightened by fearful or out-of-control thinking. Three questions can enable us to realistically assess a situation.

- Is this a real tiger or paper tiger?
- Is this problem temporary?
- Is this situation permanent?

Real tiger or paper tiger
We were designed to run from tigers or whatever predators existed in the land of your ancestors. The thoughtful, wise part of our brain shuts down when under attack because our entire focus is on escape. We are not supposed to negotiate with predators. And we can't be empathetic in these times, because we are not supposed to ask the tiger how it feels while it attacks us. Hear this clearly: During the worst moments of stress, humans cannot optimally draw from 2 of our most innate resilience tools, thoughtfulness and empathy toward others.

We can guide our children to first ask themselves, "Is this a real tiger or a paper tiger?" If the situation isn't physically dangerous the answer is "paper tiger." Once we realize we are safe, we can regain our thinking capacities and better connect to others.

Is this problem temporary?
When highly stressed, we might imagine a problem will have far-reaching, long-lasting, even catastrophic consequences. Breathe. Ask yourself, "How will I feel in a month or even a week?" If the answer is, "I won't be as upset about this," then offer self-reassurance: "This too shall pass."

Is this situation permanent?
Sometimes people feel anxious about losing the good fortune they have had. This expectation of impending loss or failure reinforces a lack of control. Instead, we want our children to remind themselves that good things *can* be long-lasting if they create circumstances where positive things come to them. In other words, when they understand they have earned their circumstances, rather than having been lucky, they will feel a greater sense of control in their life.

Comprehensive coping plan for children, adolescents, and you

A comprehensive stress-reduction plan should include strategies that would prepare us to

- Accurately assess the stressor (as previously described).
- Effectively problem-solve to address issues driving the stress.
- Utilize exercise, good nutrition, proper sleep, and effective relaxation to produce the physical state essential for the resilient mind to manage stress.
- Manage emotions in a healthy way. Some strategies should offer healthy ways to avoid experiencing every feeling and others should enable us to express and release emotions.
- Commit to contribute to others' lives. This gives people a sense of meaning and purpose and helps them understand that their well-being matters to others.

The following plan has 10 points to implement the aforementioned strategies. Though they are numbered, the 10 points are not meant to go in order, but, rather, each can be drawn from when appropriate. *Building Resilience in Children and Teens: Giving Kids Roots and Wings* offers a deep dive into activities and actions in each category.

Category 1: Tackling the problem

Point 1: Identify and then address the problem. If we address the problem, we reduce the source of stress. One strategy is to name the problem and then break it into smaller pieces, using lists or timelines designed to facilitate tackling one issue at a time. This helps us to reframe problems from being mountains too overwhelmingly high to climb into smaller hills we can more easily scale. As we reach the top of each hill, it becomes easier to imagine conquering the mountain.

Point 2: Avoid stress when possible. The most efficient thing we can do is choose to avoid being triggered by a source of stress. If, for example, there is a person who bullies in school, your child should turn to an adult to create a safe environment. If a person who bullies lives in the community and only harasses your child when they walk on the street, plan a new route.

Point 3: Let some things go. People should conserve energy to address problems they can fix. This builds their sense of control rather than reinforcing the sense of inadequacy, frustration, and anger that comes from trying to fix an issue they cannot affect. The serenity prayer captures this point.

> *"Grant me the serenity to accept the things I cannot change; the courage to change the things I can; and the wisdom to know the difference."*

Category 2: Taking care of my body

Point 4: The power of exercise. Stress hormones prevent our ability to focus. Our body senses a "tiger" may be preparing to pounce, and our anxiety builds if we have no plan to escape. Exercise is tightly linked to emotional well-being and positively affects stress, anxiety, and depression. Perhaps this is because it communicates to our bodies, "I've outrun the tiger and I am safe!"

Point 5: Active relaxation. To regain the focus needed to manage stress, we need to quiet the mind. Deep breathing is the portal to focused relaxation. It is the starting point to gain focus and therefore the anchor of yoga, meditation, mindfulness, and martial arts. We teach: *"You can flip the switch from being worried to relaxed if you know how to breathe yourself into a calm state."* Many digital apps and online videos teach effective breathing techniques.

Point 6: Eat well. Good nutrition creates a healthy body and clear mind. Help your child understand: *"Good nutrition keeps us alert and our mood steady. Junk food creates highs and lows in our energy level and interferes with our stable moods. Eating fruits, vegetables, lean proteins, and whole grains keeps us focused longer."*

Point 7: Sleep well. Rest is essential to stress management. People do not sleep well if they have too much stimulation in their bedrooms or keep irregular hours. People rest more easily when they resolve or release problems (see point 9) before bedtime or actively choose to set them aside before settling in for the night.

Category 3: Dealing with emotions

Point 8: Take instant vacations. Sometimes the best way to lower stress is to "disappear" to a more relaxing place. We can access our imagination and choose to focus on our interests rather than problems. Reading for pleasure is a proven way to escape thoughts and feelings because it immerses us in other realities. This strategy is key to drug prevention because it offers a healthy way to disengage from problems and lessens the need for an unhealthy quick fix. Our imaginations are always with us and a book can be in our bag or downloaded onto tablets or our phones.

Point 9: Release emotional tension. We need to express emotions rather than let them build (see Chapter 12). This includes connecting to others and letting go of feelings through spoken, written, and various creative expression. We can express emotions with anything that completes this thought, "I _____ it out!" Strategies that can fill in the blank include prayed, laughed, talked, cried, drew, sung, danced, rapped, wrote, or screamed.

Category 4: Making the world better helps you feel better

Point 10: Contribute. Contribution to others pays off by building stronger communities and families and by helping us gain a fuller sense of personal meaning. Critically, it may help people feel more comfortable turning to others during a time of need, and that ultimately could be the decisive factor in managing stress.

Stress management in a crisis

A stress-management plan requires an intentional, thoughtful approach. But thinking is not our strong suit when we are highly anxious or stressed. This is how to get started.

1. **Exercise first.** Our stress hormones communicate "RUN" to our bodies and we can't access our thinking powers while ignoring our

instincts. Exercise settles the brain by communicating back to our stress hormones, "I'm listening to you, I'm escaping."

2. **Breathe.** Breathing deeply and methodically turns on the relaxed nervous system. It calms the body and activates the mind. It communicates to the stress hormones, "I am safe. If I were under attack, do you think I'd be breathing with this much control?"

3. **Now, think.** Now that the stress hormones are used up and the relaxed nervous system has been activated, problem-solving can begin. Start with a self-reminder: "I am not in danger." Once the brain senses safety, you can build a solution.

4. **Express emotions** in a healthy way (see point 9).

Resources

Building Resilience in Children and Teens: Giving Kids Roots and Wings has 5 chapters focused on enabling you to support your children and teens to build their stress management and coping skill sets.

The Center for Parent and Teen Communication through **https://parentandteen** **.com** offers free practical strategies to strengthen family connections and foster youth prepared to thrive.

Parentandteen.com helps adults learn to guide youth to build their stress-management skills. It offers an interactive stress-management plan that guides young people to build a range of stress-management strategies. They will be able to download their self-designed plan as a PDF. (It does not substitute for the protective power of human relationships nor replace professional guidance.)

- https://parentandteen.com/category/health-prevention/helping-teens-cope
- https://parentandteen.com/teen-stress-management-plan

CHAPTER 20

Resilience 201: Preparing Our Children to Live in an Uncertain World

We cannot control all the waves our children will ride but can prepare them to handle them and to thrive. Modeling how we respond to the unforeseeable elements of our lives and manage inevitable frustrations shows our children how they, too, might handle uncertainty.

Uncertainty takes a toll on our physical and psychological well-being. We have a deep-seated biological understanding of how to react to imminent danger—the real tigers. Our fight-or-flight response transforms our bodies to survive. Our hearts race to pump more blood to our muscles so we can run, and our pupils dilate to see everything that might hinder our escape. However, we're not wired to deal efficiently with the tiger who *might* be lurking in the grass. We must remain vigilant and prepared to respond if a tiger does suddenly lunge. That state of constant preparedness fuels emotional discomfort and generates unhealthy hormones that harm our bodies. We can limit that harm if we raise children prepared to manage uncertainty.

Preparing for Adolescence

Adolescents work hard to gain a deeper understanding of how our society functions. In uncertain times or when our society is dysfunctional, it can take a large toll on their sense of security or how they view their future. We cannot shield them from challenges, but we can help them build their resilience in uncertain times, largely by surrounding themselves with positive human supports and seeking accurate information.

Shaping Your Lifelong Bond

Life will continue to have moments of insecurity. When your child learns that we make safe havens within our homes to support one another, it will influence how they shape the households they will create as adults. It will also likely ensure that you will be mutually reliant on one another in future uncertain times.

Make the Unpredictable Predictable

We exercise our children's resilience muscles if they notice a pattern in how we manage uncertainty. This chapter offers many strategies to manage uncertainty, but let's underscore 3 key points here.

- In our own most vulnerable moments, we draw nearer to those we love. This doesn't eliminate uncertainty but ensures that a strengthening experience accompanies challenging times.
- Anticipate disruptions whenever possible to minimize surprises. If there are circumstances likely to get in the way of routines, create alternate plans.
- Explain the circumstances causing the disruptions. Don't assume the worst. Instead, state what you know, what you don't, and your strategy to learn more. Knowledge is power and shifts the "tiger hidden in the grass" into something you can see.

Create a safe haven

As discussed in Chapter 1, we can create sanctuaries within our homes when the world is uncertain. We occasionally display our worst selves during stressful times, but long-standing security takes hold when we realize we are still cared about and worthy not only of love but of compassion and forgiveness.

A safe haven should be a place where we can remain calm, thoughtful, and reflective. Limit the barrage of media-driven information while having planned check-ins with credible sources of information. Unplug from social media, while staying connected to a trusted support network of friends and relatives.

Be a source of calm for others

Our minds sometimes imagine the worst-case scenario in moments of uncertainty. A reassuring and caring presence makes all the difference in slowing our minds as they race toward catastrophic thought. Chapter 3 covered co-regulation in detail, including the fact that we are only sources of calm when our minds are settled. This takes resolve and commitment to first access your own self-regulation strategies. It pays off because our children benefit from seeing how we become calm as much as they benefit from our calming presence.

Focus on reality

Anxiety is often fueled by our minds racing to worst-case scenarios. Catastrophic thinking activates our stress responses and interferes with our ability to take actions rooted in thoughtful, reality-based plans. Catastrophic thinking sounds like a dialogue in your head that is telling a story about how things will only worsen. Children learn how to control their internal dialogue from you if you talk out loud about how you understand—and then control—the connections between inaccurate thoughts and uncomfortable feelings. For example, when you feel your mind racing, you might say, "My imagination just took hold of my thoughts, and I suddenly became worried about something that wasn't even happening, but it still made me feel panicky. Once I realized those thoughts were only in my head, I took a deep breath, and stopped them. Now I can focus on reality and what actually is happening." In Chapter 21, we'll discuss how to alter our thinking patterns once we realize our thoughts are getting away from us.

Focus on what you can do

Resilience is about stretching into new territory you didn't think you could handle. Gaining strength. Being prepared for challenges but also being committed to relish life's joyful moments. Resilient people take control of what we can.

- When we view problems as insurmountable, we feel powerless. But even if we can't solve a problem entirely, we can usually work on partial solutions. This reduces feeling overwhelmed and builds our resolve to take another step.

- Resilient people know when to double down on their efforts and when to conserve energy by adapting to reality. It's important to know when we can't change something and to instead focus on what we *can* do to improve circumstances.
- Even in the toughest times, create space for joy. That may mean staying present with those around you or being intentional about inviting others into your life. It may mean setting aside worries and choosing to relax, play a game, or enjoy comfort food.
- We must fill our lives with reminders that even if we can't control everything, we *do* matter to others. Contributing to others' lives gives our own lives value (see Chapter 24).

"I don't know" is an answer

You want your child to become comfortable with not knowing the answer to everything. You model this best when you're clear about what you know, what you don't, and the steps you take to learn more. When you remain calm, maintain a hopeful outlook, and demonstrate thoughtfulness, you show how to cope with uncertainty.

- Help your child stretch into being secure in not knowing but committed to learning. "You're asking great questions. I don't know the answers, but let's seek answers from places we trust. We may not get perfect answers, but we'll move closer to finding them together."
- If something is deeply concerning but solutions are not yet apparent, you might say: "When I want good information, I look to experts who have the skills and background to find the answers. I also am more likely to trust information from people who say what they know and what they're still working to figure out. I look elsewhere for information if something is really complicated, and people give me simple answers."

Maintain hope

People become despondent without hope. Do not deny realities or make promises you can't fulfill or your child may lose trust in you. But you can and should have a hopeful outlook that will empower your child to continue to take actionable steps to get through challenging times.

- Insert one of the most calming words into your discussions: "Yet" reminds us that current circumstances do not define the future. "I'll never _____!" transforms into "I haven't _____ yet." **We want children to possess a mindset that doesn't see disappointment or discomfort as permanent but instead seeks opportunities to try *yet* again.**
- Remember, young people have not *yet* had the experience to know that crises come and go. Amid a crisis, it is usually hard to see past it. Repeat what your elders likely passed down to you: "This too shall pass." Give those words more power by underscoring your unwavering presence: "And we'll get through this together."
- Reinforce there is power in leaning on others for support. Instill hope by maintaining certainty that joining with other people helps people feel better and usually creates the combined thinking power that more easily arrives at solutions.

Model self-forgiveness

In uncertain times, we rarely accomplish all we'd hope and must be satisfied with good enough. When we are intentional about self-compassion and genuine acceptance even when we don't hit the intended mark, our children learn that it's OK to give themselves a break. They'll see through your example that when we care for ourselves, we are better positioned to care for others. Remember, as discussed in Chapter 5, they'll more likely include you in the details of their lives when they've seen you as self-forgiving. It reassures them you'll offer them compassion when they need it.

Protecting children from people who exploit their insecurity

Real or not, true or false?

We are driven to understand the forces that shape our lives. This drives scientific exploration. It also motivates us to connect with others who may possess knowledge or have earned wisdom under similar circumstances. However, the human need for answers cannot always be quickly satisfied, and we can be led astray. Sometimes people offer well-intentioned misinformation. This type of information might consist of a person sharing the answers that make sense to them but that are incorrect.

But we must be especially suspicious of people who take advantage of our vulnerabilities by sharing hateful and divisive ideas. Tragically, when some people are frightened, they look for a scapegoat to blame and that too often is a group they define as different from them—as "other." Consequently, precisely when we should be drawing nearer to each other in our communities or as a nation, hatred and divisiveness rise. Part of preparing your child to be resilient in an uncertain world is to prepare them to recognize hatred masked as easy answers.

Threats and blackmail

Children and teens can be exploited, threatened, and even blackmailed by people who take advantage of the fact that uncertainty can trigger insecurity and profound anxiety. The threat of a ruined reputation will upset anyone but can destroy an adolescent who may feel their social standing defines them. There are terrifying cases of teenagers being coerced into inappropriate actions through social media and then threatened with disclosure. Tell your child that no matter how scary or threatening something might feel, you will always stand by them. Let them know that they can come to you no matter what. In exchange for their trust in you, pledge that in the worst or most uncertain of times you would never punish them for a mistake and instead would offer them unwavering support and guidance.

CHAPTER 21

Resilience 301: Becoming (More) Comfortable With Discomfort

Taking on discomfort is uncomfortable. It is made more so if the people you care about suggest you are weak or incapable because of your comfort threshold. Humans are not supposed to ignore discomfort. In fact, our feelings of discomfort are an important signal that something might be wrong. But we do want to accurately assess whether we should avoid the source of discomfort or lean into it and learn to manage it. Because dealing with challenges is part of being alive, we want to raise our children not to be hindered by the challenges they'll face and, when appropriate, to stretch into new territory. People gain confidence when they realize they can take on something they hadn't previously thought they could.

A Lighthouse Parent, like every parent, wishes they could ensure nothing but safe passages for their children. But because no parent holds that power, we instead raise them to tolerate life's distressing moments. We won't be standing alongside them during most of life's toughest moments, so we instill in them the good judgment to manage what they can and to know when their discomfort signals danger to avoid.

Preparing for Adolescence

Many adolescents worry about how they perform in different settings and how people view them. In fact, their thoughts can run away from them. You can help them control their thinking patterns so they can more comfortably evaluate and deal with challenges. Using the language of resilience, you can communicate your trust in their ability to manage challenges.

Shaping Your Lifelong Bond

Nobody wants to be seen as a problem to be solved. Rather, we want to be viewed as problem-solvers. Your adult child will invite you into their lives as a continued source of support when they know that you see them as capable of managing their own discomfort and as someone who wisely *chooses* to draw support from others.

Lend Your Calm and Model Calming Strategies

Because children sense safety and gain security from us, we build their confidence to take reasonable chances when they know *we* are comfortable. We model 2 equally important points: 1) There are times when we must respond fully to danger signals; and 2) We are intentional, and maybe even methodical, in expanding our comfort zones. Remember, if it looks too easy for you to manage a challenge, your child may feel incapable when something doesn't feel easy to them. If, on the other hand, you model the steps you take to assess and then manage a situation, they'll see that it is something they can learn. Several chapters have prepared you to offer these lessons. In Chapter 6, we underscored that modeling what it really means to be an adult doesn't mean making it look easy. In Chapters 19 and 20, we covered strategies you can pass along (and practice) to deal with uncertainty and manage stressors.

It's important that you do the hard work to get and stay calm (see Chapter 3). And make sure your unspoken signals support the words you plan to say.

To recap, when getting calm

- Remind yourself that if you know something serious is going on in your child's life it means you are trusted with their discomfort, and that is a healthy place to be as a parent.
- Trust your child will get through uncomfortable moments. Take deep breaths to prevent yourself from slipping into panic mode.
- Don't feel like you need to supply all the answers. Listening is easier *and* the best strategy. Admit if you don't yet have solutions. Express confidence you'll find them in time.
- Trust that with time and gentle guidance, your child will come to *their* solution.

When reinforcing your reliable *and helpful* presence

- Show up. Stay present. It *is* that simple.
- You'll only be helpful if your child doesn't fear losing you. Remember you can disapprove of a behavior while making it clear you fully approve of your child.
- Don't let your body language (or words) suggest their emotions are wrong or more than you can handle. For example, don't slink out of the room and never get back to the conversation.
- Don't miss the expression of strong emotions thinking they'll go away with only the passage of time.
- Don't overemphasize a problem or deny it.
- Remember, even the most intelligent or mature person who is in crisis needs to be spoken to in calm, simple language (see Chapter 11).

Keep your eye on building resilience

As you support your child to build resilience in the face of discomfort, it can be helpful to consider the 7 Cs framework.

The 7 Cs of Resilience	Elevating Resilience
Competence	Elevate the skill sets your child possesses by reinforcing how they could be helpful to deal with the current situation. If they have not yet developed a skill set, then focus on building strategies to deal with the challenge.
Confidence	Notice what your child is already doing to manage their discomfort. Focus on the effort they're putting in rather than whether they've yet resolved an issue. This decreases anxiety about taking on a challenge because they know they don't have to solve it entirely to please you. They only need to commit to growth.
Connection	Even in the toughest moments, we show up and demonstrate our reliable presence. The only thing we can be certain of is that people are stronger when together and wiser when they support each other to find solutions.
Character	We never define our children based on our judgment of a specific behavior or their discomfort. Rather, we focus on all that is good and right about them. When our children seek a solution to a problem, we root our guidance in their existing strengths.

Contribution	People who care deeply are gifted with sensitivity and poised to make a difference in other lives. We recognize and celebrate this gift even as we help address current struggles. We remind children that as they learn to help themselves, they will better support others in the future.
Coping	We guide our children to manage uncomfortable thoughts and feelings in a positive way rather than telling them what they should not do.
Control	We recognize children as experts in their own lives. We support them to develop solutions while asking their guidance about how and where to best apply strategies that will help them lessen discomfort.

Catastrophic thinking is not reality

Sometimes our discomfort is based on false or exaggerated scenarios only playing out in our minds. As our thoughts race to the worst possible outcomes, our stress responses are activated. Our hearts quicken and our stomachs turn. Our thoughts become dysregulated, and we can find ourselves falling into despair, despite nothing having changed. Learning to control these thoughts is the first step to solution-building and resilient thinking.

Realistic thinking enables thoughtfully crafted solutions. It doesn't minimize problems but rather limits discomfort because we can learn to reframe situations and find workable solutions. The Penn Resiliency Project, headed by Martin E.P. Seligman, PhD, of the University of Pennsylvania, has conducted some of the most influential studies demonstrating the importance of changing our thinking patterns. He mentored several leading experts in resilience, including Karen Reivich, PhD. Dr Seligman, Dr Reivich, and colleagues demonstrated that children and adults can rethink a situation, shift their thinking patterns that were causing them to spiral into catastrophic thinking, and thereby restore their positive outlooks. Two of their books, *The Optimistic Child: A Proven Program to Safeguard Children Against Depression and Build Lifelong Resilience* (Martin Seligman, PhD, with Karen Reivich, PhD; Lisa Jaycox, PhD; and Jane Gillham, PhD) and *The Resilience Factor* (Karen Reivich, PhD, and Andrew Shatté, PhD) offer deep dives into how to build healthier thinking patterns. Some key points from these books are summarized in the following paragraphs:

We can "catch" our thoughts when we stop ourselves from falling into familiar thinking patterns. Catastrophic thinking sounds like a conversation in your mind about how things will only worsen. There are words that repeat in our minds and offer a clue that catastrophic thinking will begin. Words like, "If I don't _____," or "I better _____," or "Now that _____ has happened, _____ will likely happen." Catch yourself and instead say, "I am imagining this." "I am creating this worry." Breathe. Then ask, "What is *really* happening *right now*? What is *really* the worst-case scenario? What *could be* the best thing that happens, not the worst?" Reality is usually somewhere between the 2 extremes. Return to the present moment, where you can problem-solve while rooted in reality.

Model this from the time your children are young by talking out loud to help them see how inaccurate thoughts lead to uncomfortable feelings. "Wow, you wouldn't believe where my imagination just took me. It felt real but it wasn't. Once I took a deep breath, I caught myself thinking a huge problem was happening, but it wasn't! Now I'm going to focus on what I can change."

When you think your child is ready, you can teach them the following 4-step strategy:

1. Recognize negative thoughts when they begin to take over. Catch the clues when too-familiar phrases such as, "I better," "If I don't," or "I should" begin a thought. This strategy/concept is aptly called *thought catching!*
2. Stop. Ask yourself whether those thoughts are accurate. What is *really* happening?
3. Create accurate explanations when challenging situations occur. Avoid turning to self-blame.
4. Decatastrophize. Ground yourself in reality. Neither a mistake nor failure, not even others' anger or disappointment, lead to disaster when we can think through a solution.

Dr Reivich's book teaches how adults can help young people learn to catch their inner thoughts and therefore change some of the patterns of their reactions to events. The following "ABC technique" described by Dr Reivich is rooted in the cognitive techniques originated by Albert Ellis, PhD. We often focus on the **A** (activating events or "What happened?") and quickly leap to the outcome **C** (consequences or "How do you feel now?" or "What are you going to do?"). This misses the opportunity for our children to better understand the **B** connectors, the beliefs fueled by the silent *self-talk* that drives their feelings and ultimately responses. When we instead say, "What are you thinking now?" we have a better opportunity to help them learn to pause, consider their thoughts instead of their reactions, and thereby disrupt and redirect their internal dialogue.

If your child's thought patterns interfere with their well-being, speak to your pediatrician or school counselor about a referral to a cognitive behavioral therapist. Learning healthier thinking patterns can manage or even prevent discomfort.

The language of resilience

When our children experience discomfort, *we* experience discomfort. We can't shield them from all that might hurt them, but we can prepare them to handle life's tough moments. This means setting aside our instinctual need to protect them from a temporary challenge and to instead choose a strategy that prepares them to handle it. We can help them understand they can take control over their lives by managing their thoughts and feelings and creating solutions. Learning to problem-solve involves trial and error as children stretch beyond existing comfort zones. If we as parents allow ourselves to be driven by frustrations or worries, our words will express our hopelessness or fear. This will generate anxiety in our children and prevent them from gaining the confidence they need to comfortably stretch and ultimately address and resolve the source of discomfort.

Our words express how we view our children and teens and shape how they see themselves. Do we see them as vulnerable or as strong and resilient? Incapable or thoughtful and wise? When we state our desire to jump in to fix a situation, "Let me help you out," we communicate, "I don't think you can handle this." Our words must convey that we trust them to grow and ultimately manage distress.

Say This (about your child's strengths and limitations)	Not That	Because
This is a real strength of yours.	This really worked out for you.	To gain a sense of control, children need to understand their actions and skills, not luck, create good outcomes.
This is a limitation you'll need to conquer.	This is your weakness.	A "weakness" is permanent. A limitation can be overcome with proper actions.

Say This (when engaging your child's thoughtfulness)	Not That	Because
What do you think?	I think . . .	To move your child to the next step you must know their starting point. Once you begin problem-solving, they'll stop developing solutions on their own.
Tell me what you understand.	You're too young to understand.	Each person of every age has an understanding from which growth flows. If you don't start guidance from your child's initial understanding, you might deliver information they can't grasp.

Say This (about performance)	Not That	Because
It feels overwhelming. But it's not a real tiger and this can't hurt you. You'll focus better and perform better if you remember that.	If you don't do well on this test, you'll never reach your goals. If you don't play well, you'll lose your spot on the team.	High pressure stakes bring out our stress reactions, which prevent us from thinking clearly or connecting best (essential to being on a team) with others.
People are uneven, possessing both strengths and limitations. Hard work ensures you'll learn about your strengths. Some things will be more difficult for you, but real effort ensures you'll learn as much as you can.	Just work hard and you'll do well.	It isn't true that hard work always leads to a good performance. When children discover this, they'll disavow your encouragement and give up. Instead, they should know we get better (not perfect) at anything we apply ourselves to.
You worked hard and it paid off with a good result.	You are so good at _____.	When children are told what they are good at, they become fixed in the belief it's all they excel in. We want children to learn they influence outcomes with their *effort*. This reinforces a growth mindset.[1]

---

1. Dweck CS. *Mindset: The New Psychology of Success.* 2nd ed. Ballantine Books; 2016.

You earned it.	You got lucky.	Children must learn that they have control over their actions so they can be driven to take the next step.
I know you feel you were treated unfairly. What might you have done to have contributed to it not working out the way you wanted?	It was the teacher's/coach's fault. You didn't do anything wrong.	Even in difficult interactions, we must learn that we can limit the discomfort by controlling what we can. This can either be our own actions or how we react to others' actions.

Say This (about problem-solving or solution-building)	Not That	Because
How would you solve this problem?	Let me help you with that.	We must show trust in our children's growing capacity rather than communicate we'll handle it.
What do you think is the best way to solve this? How can I support your plan?	I'll handle this for you.	We need our children to brainstorm solutions them-selves—to stretch. That's hard work they may not begin if there is an easy way out.
Take one step at a time. When you've accomplished something small, you'll know you can succeed and feel less overwhelmed.	Just get started.	Starting feels overwhelming. Taking steps one at a time lays out a path.

Say This (about a bad experience)	Not That	Because
This must feel awful. In time, it will hurt less. And you'll learn how to handle a similar problem if it comes up again.	It's not that bad.	Children talk to us if we understand how deeply they feel. If we belittle or diminish their feelings, they'll stop sharing.
You'll get through this.	I'll protect you.	Children need to know they have the power within themselves to heal. Part of their power is receiving support and guidance from others. If their parents handle it all, they'll never earn trust in their own abilities.
This awful feeling will pass. It hurts now, but you'll feel a bit better over time.	This is terrible.	People need hope and a reminder that their discom-fort will lessen.

Say This (about emotional distress)	Not That	Because
Your sensitivity might be your greatest strength. So many people will benefit from it. Your challenge will be to learn how to care so much without it causing so much personal discomfort.	You're too sensitive.	Sensitive people couldn't turn off their feelings if they wanted to, nor should they. They must see it as a strength, but one they need to protect with self-care and reflection.
I am so proud of how deeply you think. Your challenge is to be sure that your thoughts are accurate. Sometimes thoughtful people create worries in their imagination. Catch those uncomfortable thoughts and remind yourself you'll be able to handle what is really going on. Your thoughtfulness is exactly how you'll problem-solve.	You worry too much.	Children can't turn off thinking, but they can alter their thought patterns. Sometimes worrying is a sign of great intelligence and sensitivity. It should be recognized as a strength we need to harness.

Most Critically, Say This	Not That	Because
I don't think you're ready yet. What do you think you have to do to become ready to handle this?	No.	Our children should always know that we see them as developing beings. That gives them the confidence and the drive to stretch.

"Yet": A Word That Shows Change Is Possible and Discomfort Is Temporary

None of us are good at everything. Children might feel defeated when they can't grasp a school subject or demoralized when they feel limited on the athletic field. And sometimes life hands us challenges we don't think we'll ever get past. Children sometimes feel as though they'll never fit in socially or figure out how to handle problems as easily as the adults in their lives do.

Self-defeating thoughts often begin with words such as, "I never" or "I can't." As previously suggested, help your child catch those thoughts and then insert the word "yet" into their internal dialogue. "I can't solve this problem" becomes, "I haven't *yet* solved this problem." With this hope, now your child can free their mind to create an action plan.

We want children to develop a mindset that doesn't accept failure as permanent. We want them to accept that nobody is good at everything or fits in socially in every situation. All of us are works in progress. Setbacks are *opportunities* to try yet again. Limitations are challenges they've not *yet* learned to minimize or work around entirely.

CHAPTER 22

Resilience 401: Framing Help-Seeking as a Strength

Turning to another person and asking for support is the ultimate act of resilience. It is a sign of inner strength to know that you deserve to feel better and an act of self-confidence to take the steps to get yourself what you need. Children of Lighthouse Parents will more naturally possess this inner strength and self-confidence because they have been raised in an environment where mutual reliance is celebrated. They have learned that good times become joyous when shared and to turn to others to help weather tough moments.

Preparing for Adolescence

It is never too early to build the foundation for a healthy relationship with help-seeking. Many parents need to work through their own conflicting feelings on mental and behavioral health services as well as the feelings of failure they experience when their child is struggling. Working through this before a crisis presents will make for a much smoother experience with help-seeking in childhood or adolescence.

Shaping Your Lifelong Bond

People never outgrow the need for support. Loved ones and friends will always be the foundation of support. However, professionals can offer critical support in challenging times. You want your adult child to come to you in these difficult moments, and they are more likely to do so if they know you have a healthy view of help-seeking. They will also be more comfortable sharing their future struggles if they know you always see their strengths.

Turning to Others as a Source of Strength

Strength. Courage. Bravery. These seem like characteristics we'd like to emulate. Many of us may have been raised to think that quiet independence—going it alone and without complaints—was the definition of strength. Courage was often portrayed as defying one's self-protective instincts. Bravery was characterized as confronting problems that might humble or destroy others alone. The problem is that many people were not taught from where to source and renew their strength. Consequently, turning to others—undoubtedly the source of human strength—was too often mistakenly seen as weakness.

Modeling help-seeking

While we will focus on seeking professional support in this chapter, most support often comes from family, friends, and community members with whom we share our lives. It is with these people that we create good times and share resources in lean times. It is in communities that we join in social action to share our concerns and join in prayer or reflection to summon courage.

When we turn to others, our children learn that strong people are fueled by human connection. Make it known when you seek advice from others. This will normalize help-seeking as an accepted part of your family culture. If you seek professional support, you can share how it benefits you without needing to discuss any personal details. The imperative of human connection as a source of human resilience and thriving was covered in Chapter 18. The remainder of this chapter is about turning to professional services when appropriate.

Working through your feelings about mental and emotional health services

You can't predict when you might need to speak to your child about why they will benefit from professional support. You'll want them to engage positively with the support rather than feel ashamed for receiving it. If you have mixed feelings about mental health and social support services, it's important to work through your ambivalence now. Children are highly sensitive to what you are feeling, and if you do not feel positively about the benefit of support, it may make them resistant to seeking help.

Many parents have high regard for support services but see it as a personal failure when their *own* children or teens need support. Let's explore this so you can move past it. If your child senses that their seeking professional support is somehow letting you down or making you feel bad about yourself, they will reject treatment. Your child's struggles are not your failure! Parents cannot prevent their children from experiencing problems. Loving parents stand by their children when they do have problems and get them the support they deserve. Involving others who can help is a responsible and deeply loving act. Move beyond self-blame for your own sake and as an initial step to having your child comfortably accept support.

Framing help-seeking

To move past any shame or guilt, you may have to unlearn the scripts in your mind associated with help-seeking. These thoughts may reiterate what people have said to you. Though these words weren't offered with harmful intent, they may have suggested our distress was rooted in something about us that we needed fixed or that they would go away with a healthy dose of denial.

Say This (about seeking help)	Not That	Because
A strong person chooses to reach out to others.	A strong person handles tough times.	We must frame help-seeking as an act of strength.
It'll take time. But the support you'll get from those who care about you will help you heal and help you build on your own strength.	Just get past it.	Time does heal. But we should be actively seeking support during that time, not tucking away our emotions.

Sometimes the strongest thing a person can do is to seek professional help.	Strong people move on.	It is an act of bravery to know that you have more than you can handle. It allows you to be your best self; a person who moves on has not taken a step to resolve a problem or regain strength.
You deserve to feel better.	You need help!	The word "need" implies a deficit that must be filled. It can be experienced as negatively judgmental. "Deserve" is a positively judgmental word. It implies that there's something valuable about you and that you have earned extra attention.
You deserve to learn to manage the fullness of your emotions. I am so proud of how intensely you feel. Your challenge is to learn to manage all of those feelings so you can benefit from them without them taking a toll on you.	You need help.	We wish our children had no discomfort. But that is the toll humans pay for caring, sensitivity, and sometimes just for paying attention. Taking a strength-based approach will help your child feel empowered about managing their emotions. "You need help" sounds like you see them as broken. It also might be spoken with an angry rather than supportive tone.

Notice distress signals

Children may not tell us when they are distressed because they can't sort out their own feelings, are ashamed of what they feel, or think they spare us by holding their feelings inside. It is helpful when our children tell us what they feel, but we must remain attentive to the following unspoken signals:

- **Sudden changes in behavior** like refusing to follow rules or a radical change in peer group.
- All children can be moody, but **prolonged irritability** is a distress signal. Depressed adults admit to sadness or feeling down and may lack energy. They feel hopeless and have changes in their eating, sleeping, or hygiene patterns. This may be true for many depressed adolescents and children, but nearly half are irritable instead of withdrawn and may act out with rage.

- **Excessive worry,** inability to focus, difficulty participating in school, or discomfort engaging in social activities can signal anxiety.
- **Frequent aches and pains,** including headaches, dizziness, bellyaches, and chest pain may be signs of emotional stress. Children (and many adults) lack insight into the connection between their emotions and their bodies' responses. Health professionals will consider an underlying illness, while helping your child understand healthy people can experience physical discomfort when stressed.
- Notice signs of **exhaustion** or **difficulty waking up** in time for school. Some children have sleep disturbances when distressed.
- **Changes in school performance** can signal distress. Just as adults' work performance declines with stress, children may find it difficult to focus on schoolwork.

Never belittle your child's verbal or nonverbal signals of distress as "only attention seeking." If your child is seeking attention, give it. They'll be relieved they don't have to handle their distress alone.

Guiding your child to feel good about professional support

How you frame the help-seeking process can make the critical difference toward your child's attitude about professional support and therefore the likelihood of its success. The following suggestions come from decades of experience connecting children and families to support services. They answer many of the asked and unasked questions on children's and adolescent's minds regarding professional support. If you are still working through your own ambivalence about professional help, read the suggestions as if they were me speaking directly to you.

These suggestions try to make 3 things clear.

- Professional guidance can be helpful, and there are people who focus on supporting young people because of how much they care about them.
- Emotional discomfort is treatable, and people who have difficult times often possess great strengths like sensitivity.
- Your child will not be on this journey alone; you will stand by their side, and your relationship will become healthier and stronger.

Let them know they will not be alone

Some people fear that by getting professional help they will lose supportive relationships with family, friends, teachers, school counselors, clergy, or coaches. Naturally, they'd rather keep their existing close relationships. We must tell our children that seeking professional help does not mean giving up other critical relationships. Family and friends remain the key supports in their life. In fact, because they'll learn to manage stress, their other relationships may be strengthened.

Young people who struggle may fear that they've "messed everything up" in their important relationships. Why? Because humans often push friends and family away during times of extreme distress. Ironically, they do so precisely because they feel secure enough to reveal their most uncomfortable thoughts and feelings. It is important to state that you clearly understand their behavior reflects that they are going through something. You'll always stand by them. And a major benefit of professional support is that family relationships can be repaired and restored.

Make it clear that treatment can work

Many children may wonder, "How can it help? Why bother." It may be hard for children in distress to know they might ever feel better. Let them understand that what they are currently experiencing can be temporary and professional guidance can help them navigate their feelings. Explain that professionals have spent years learning how to be most effective and that researchers have developed approaches that work. If you know people who have benefitted from support, tell your children, without sharing specific details.

Underscore that time invested will pay off

Anxious children and teens may worry that time spent in counseling will make them fall behind in other areas. Anxiety itself may make it difficult for them to be convinced otherwise because they will have trouble calming themselves enough to hear your words. Calmly reinforce that their mental well-being is top priority. The investment in learning to reduce their spent energy in worrying will create time by increasing their efficiency and focus.

Reinforce that seeking treatment is an act of strength

Sometimes people get down on themselves because they can't "handle" their own problems, worrying that going for support means they are weak or even "crazy." A strength-based approach can change how they see themselves. Your unwavering knowledge of who they really are, beyond the challenges they may experience or the behaviors they may *temporarily* display, will give them the confidence to move forward.

It is courageous to clearly state, "I don't feel OK right now, and I want to feel better." This act of self-awareness and self-advocacy is both insightful and an act of strength. Strong people know when they are not their best selves, are capable of feeling better, deserve to feel better, and will take actionable steps to feel better.

Acknowledge that many people have challenges

Many people who endure emotional challenges retreat into themselves feeling their experience is so unique that nobody could help or fully understand them. Help your child understand all people have occasional struggles and that professionals will have experience with young people with similar challenges. Simultaneously empower your child by explaining that although emotional challenges are similar, each person's story is unique and they can help the professional to guide them most usefully by sharing their thoughts, feelings, and experiences.

Relationships with professionals are special

Some young people worry about being embarrassed by a professional or assume they will be pitied. We can help them understand that professionals commit their lives to supporting young people and have gone through years of training to be able to do so. They know that circumstances in children's lives can make it hard growing up and they do not judge them. Youth-serving professionals *choose* to work with children because they care for and respect young people. In fact, many of them serve in the field because they knew a child or teen who needed support (or struggled themselves while growing up), so they are committed to improving the lives of young people. They do care, but empathy is about seeing someone else's perspective and trying to understand what they must feel; it is not pity. If your child needs to relate to this experience, remind them that they have learned that giving back to others can feel good. This may make it easier for them to believe that the person offering them support has chosen a career of service and feels good about being able to help others.

Professionals honor privacy

Your child may say, "I don't want everybody to know my business." Help them realize that professionals are legally obligated to honor privacy. Let them know that you will honor the privacy in their relationship with the professional. Clarify that because you will always support them, you hope to know as much as they choose to share. This is another opportunity to underscore the centrality of your relationship while clearly stating that you are happy they have another trusted adult in their life.

Professionals support you

Your child may feel that existing supportive relationships are all they need. Your child may ask, "Why can't I just talk to you?" Or your child may rather just talk to friends, thinking, "They know what I'm going through better than any adult does." They need to understand how important it can be to talk to a professional who wants to hear about your feelings but whom you never have to worry about disappointing, hurting, or making angry. Relationships with friends and family are critical, but they want to protect you and you may worry about damaging your relationship. Help-seeking is an "and," not an "or." Professional guidance does not replace support from close relationships. The professional is an extra person in their life with specialized training to support your child.

Counseling builds on your strengths

Your child may think, "I'll figure out my own problems. How could someone who doesn't know what I've experienced or am feeling fix it?" Help your child understand that professionals encourage them to use skills they possess while guiding them to build new ones. Counseling offers information and strategies that can help them make good decisions, work through challenges, and manage uncomfortable feelings. Ultimately, they will solve their own problems but will be supported to do so with new skills.

Finding the right professional

Let your child know that it is important to find the right fit to best support them. This may mean meeting with some people and deciding together who is likely to be most helpful. Start with recommendations from someone you *and your child* already trust. See Resources for professional organizations that can aid your search for the best treatment for your child.

Your role while your child is receiving professional guidance

You remain the greatest source of security for your child regardless of a professional's involvement. Your unwavering presence reinforces that you will stand beside them now and long after this problem is in the rearview mirror. Remind your child that you know this problem will pass. Help them reframe their thinking though the power of a single word. "I'll never feel better again" becomes "I haven't **yet** learned how to feel better."

Keep realistic goals. You want your child to be more comfortable and always safe. You don't expect them to be perfect, just to build the inner strength to lead a satisfying and meaningful life. If it is participation in unwise behaviors that is your greatest concern, be prepared to learn the root causes driving those behaviors. You are likely to find your caring and sensitive child hiding behind the behaviors and will learn that managing their feelings is the first step to addressing their behaviors.

Strong Feelings Now Lead to a Strong Adulthood Later

It's painful to see your child in distress. But distress is a sign of sensitivity and strong feelings. You've raised a person who cares deeply! This predicts they will flourish later. People with strong feelings and deep sensitivity make trusted friends, caring life partners, reliable colleagues, and engaged, loving parents.

It is admittedly hard to feel so fully, but that doesn't mean that the feelings don't have value on the path to a rich adulthood. Your child is at the point in their journey when they must learn to manage the complexity of their feelings. If asked, they'd likely trade away that sensitivity now just to feel better. Guide them to understand that when they do learn to manage the richness of their feelings, they will be rewarded through life. And so many others will benefit from their presence.

Resources

Your child's school counselor and teachers, your pediatric health clinicians, and clergy remain primary sources of information about local mental, emotional, and behavioral health services. Following are 4 professional organizations that can assist you in finding a local licensed provider:

The American Psychological Association (APA)
https://www.apa.org
> The APA has a mission to promote the advancement, communication, and application of psychological science and knowledge to benefit society

and improve lives. They offer a wide variety of resources to help people understand the forces that have an impact on psychological health.

The APA offers a tool to "find the right psychologist for you" at https://locator.apa.org.

The American Academy of Child and Adolescent Psychiatry (AACAP)

https://www.aacap.org

The AACAP has a mission that states: To promote the healthy development of children, adolescents, and families through advocacy, education, and research. They offer rich resources to help families understand varied psychiatric conditions.

The AACAP offers a tool, the "Child and Adolescent Psychiatrist Finder," at https://www.aacap.org/AACAP/Families_Youth/CAP_Finder/AACAP/Families_and_Youth/Resources/CAP_Finder.aspx.

The American Counseling Association (ACA)

https://www.counseling.org

The ACA has a mission to promote the professional development of counselors, advocate for the profession, and ensure ethical, culturally inclusive practices that protect those using counseling services.

The ACA offers a tool to find a national certified counselor in your area at https://www.nbcc.org/search/counselorfind.

The American Association for Marriage and Family Therapy (AAMFT)

https://www.aamft.org

Marriage and family therapists are trained in psychotherapy and family systems and licensed to diagnose and treat mental and emotional disorders within the context of marriage, couples, and family systems. Their site will help you consider when individual versus family therapy may best serve your child and family.

The AAMFT offers a tool to find a marriage and family therapist in your area at https://www.therapistlocator.net.

CHAPTER 23

What It Means to Thrive: Raising Children Prepared to Do and Be Good

The ability to recover or rebound from challenges—resilience—is an essential strength we hope to develop in our children. We trust that when equipped with the resilience to weather tough times, children will also be able to experience the good times more fully and perhaps even with deeper appreciation. But our goal is loftier than to raise just resilient children. It is to raise children prepared to *flourish*. To *thrive*. But what does that mean?

People who thrive are successful. But being "successful" in the most meaningful sense does not refer to materialistic possessions but, rather, to be able to draw from the richness life offers. People who possess critical strengths of character are more likely to get the most out of life and to contribute to those around them. Part of what it means to be successful, therefore, is to be good and to do good—to care for and about others.

To be clear, you also want your child to achieve in traditional ways (academic, economic), and certainly you want them to experience happiness. Caring for and about others does not replace material accomplishments or academic achievement, but it puts them into perspective. Caring for and about others does not diminish your child's own desires for happiness, but it may mean that they will experience genuine contentment when doing what is right, generous, and fair.

Preparing for Adolescence

Our children thrive when we support them to build strong values and to be their best selves. We do this by noticing their core goodness and building on *their* strengths. This creates a strong internal moral compass that will guide them through adolescence and beyond.

Shaping Your Lifelong Bond

Key to helping children learn to thrive is modeling for them how an adult lives up to their own values. You don't do this by pretending it is easy or without struggle. You model as best you can and then discuss the hard work it takes to live up to your values. This open communication will be a lifelong template for you and your adult child as they too struggle to do the hard work of trying to be a good person.

What Is a Character Strength?

Angela Duckworth, PhD, cofounder and chief scientist of Character Lab, speaks of character as "everything we do to help other people as well as ourselves." Character Lab turns scientific discoveries about the mindsets and skills that develop character into actionable guidance. It describes 3 character strength categories: strengths of heart, strengths of mind, and strengths of will. I suggest going to their site (see Resources) to explore the playbooks to help your child build each of these sets of strengths.

- **Strengths of heart** are the "giving" strengths. They enable us to reach, support, and make a difference for others. They include the capacity to care for others and to experience empathy for them. Our essential kindness can fuel our generosity (see Chapter 26) and drive a sense of purpose within us (see Chapter 24).
- **Strengths of mind** allow us to thoughtfully reason and think creatively. These strengths include wise decision-making capabilities coupled with the curiosity and creativity that allow us to consider solutions beyond our existing comfort zone. Intellectual humility prevents us from being

entrenched in our own ideas and to recognize our own limitations (see Chapter 27). Because intellectual humility allows us to be open to others' ideas, it is a foundation of growth.

- **Strengths of will** are the strengths that make it more likely to achieve goals that are important to us. Character Lab describes these as the "doing" strengths. They include a growth mindset (see Chapter 25) and grit, a concept aptly summarized by the subtitle of Dr Duckworth's deeply influential book, *Grit: The Power of Passion and Perseverance*.

Richard Lerner, PhD, who leads the Institute for Applied Research in Youth Development, has stated that "character is about doing the right thing even when no one else is looking." Although there is not a precise recipe to build character in our children, research offers critical insights into character building, demonstrates the importance of character to human flourishing, and underscores the irreplaceable role of adults in helping to shape children's character.

There are many character strengths that enable us to live richer, fuller lives and to be better poised to contribute to others. I encourage you to use the resources listed at the end of this chapter to explore character strengths in greater depth and to consider how to support your child in developing them. In the next few chapters, we focus on a few character strengths while considering your critical role in helping your child develop their character.

How to Support Character Development in Your Child

You play an irreplaceable role in supporting your child to shape themself into the person you know they can become. You can't tell them what to believe in or insist on what they do, but as a lighthouse you remain a beacon that gives them direction. And the way you do this is not only by having a dream of who you want them to be, but rather knowing who they really are—and have always been, as discussed in Chapter 7. When you understand who they are at their core, even when they question themselves or are behaving badly, they can always look to you as a reminder of who they are at their best.

Support your child to develop character strengths

Marvin Berkowitz, PhD, director of the Center for Character and Citizenship at The University of Missouri–St. Louis, has spent decades exploring how to develop moral character strengths in our children. He suggests following the DENIM model, which stands for *demandingness, empowerment, nurturance, induction,* and *modeling.* This set of behaviors, all well supported by parenting research, can serve as your guide as you support your child's character development.

Demandingness

Young people respond to our expectations and therefore we should set them high but within reach. It is our job to make it easier to meet those expectations by offering them needed resources and guidance. This ties into the importance of knowing your child. We are all uneven and children are at different places in their development. If you set expectations at a level your child is not yet able to meet, they will feel as though they are failing. Instead, root your expectations in what you know they can do as their best self and encourage them to stretch a bit. (Remember, we are not merely speaking of their best academic achievement or their best on a playing field but, most importantly, their best in terms of their moral selves.) Dr Berkowitz emphasizes, "We must provide resources to help them have a chance—not a guarantee, just a chance—of meeting our high expectations. We want them to know that while it is important to meet our expectations, they also need to feel safe to fail." He goes on to explain that it is safe for your child to fail when they don't have to ever worry about losing your love or support.

Empowerment

As we covered in our discussion on discipline, a goal of healthy development is for children to become increasingly comfortable with independence and to gain an increasing sense of control over their lives. They must know their opinions matter enough to be heard and honored. Therefore, as we discuss moral values, they must have the opportunity to discuss and reflect upon their values. **When children are heard they feel empowered.** We can create safe spaces where emotions can be expressed, thinking can be developed, and moral values can be clarified.

We must also support our children's ability to live to the values they care about. This may involve helping them to develop the skill sets that empower them to follow through on the values their inner voice suggests they should follow even it means doing something different than peers. As our children enter adolescence, part of empowerment is creating room for them to make their own decisions and to learn from natural consequences, as discussed in Chapter 16.

Nurturance

Our unconditional and unwavering love gives children the security to develop their own values. Your child's security is largely rooted in knowing that no behavior would cause them to lose your love. As we discussed in Chapter 16, you can reject a behavior while still fully accepting the child. Your child should know that it is because of your love for them that you are so committed to them developing into a good person. Remember that your words matter, but it is your actions that will be trusted more. Even in disappointment, convey with your continued presence and attention to *their* emotions that you would never give up on them.

Induction

"Induction" sounds like a technical term but is a core element of good parenting. It is about how we let children know what we feel about their behavior. According to Merriam-Webster, induction is defined as "the act of causing or bringing on or about." In this case, you "bring about" moral character development by letting your child know how you feel. Dr Berkowitz suggests the following 3 actions:

- *Clearly tell your child how you feel about what they did.* Focus on their action ("I am so frustrated with how you …"); don't generalize it to them as a person. "Frustrated" is how what they *did* made you feel.
- *Explain why you feel the way you do in language they can understand.* ("I am so frustrated with how you ___because ___"). The "because" is key; this is how they know why you feel as you do. Further, it emphasizes that while what they did created the feeling, your view of them as a person has not changed.
- *Highlight the effects of their behavior and how what they did made someone else feel.* ("I am frustrated with how you let your brother down by teasing him about something you know he really worries about. In this family we support each other. Instead, your brother is crying because of how you made him feel.") This last point underscores what moral behavior should—and should not—look like and how each of our actions can affect others.

Modeling

How we model behavior serves as a blueprint for children of what adults are supposed to look like and is likely more meaningful than our words. Dr Berkowitz notes, "It is not a matter of deciding to be a role model. We are all role models, whether we like it or not. There is no off switch. Rather, the only choice is whether to be a good role model or not." You don't have to be perfect. You create real opportunities for discussion when your child notices your actions and you speak about the internal wrestling we all do to control our impulses. You can contribute to your child's moral development with meaningful discussions about why you do what you do and the steps you take to hold yourself to your values. If you make it look too easy, they won't be able to imagine getting there.

Resources

Center for Character and Citizenship engages in research, education, and advocacy to foster the development of character, democratic citizenship, and a civil society. Its site includes a parent toolbox and resources for communities and teachers. https://characterandcitizenship.org

Character.org is composed of educators, researchers, and business and civic leaders who care deeply about the vital role that character will play in our future. Its worldwide network empowers people of all ages to practice and model core values that shape our hearts, minds, and choices. It provides resources for developing character in families, schools, and organizations. https://character.org

Character Lab turns scientific discoveries about the mindsets and skills that develop character into actionable advice for parents and teachers. On this website, you'll find playbooks, organized by character strength, with information and activities based on rigorous research studies on how to model and reinforce character strengths. https://characterlab.org

The Center for Parent and Teen Communication offers practical strategies rooted in what is known to work to strengthen family connections and build youth prepared to thrive. It includes content on strategies to build character strengths. https://parentandteen.com

Making Caring Common Project. Its stated vision is "a world in which children learn to care about others and the common good, treat people well day to day, come to understand and seek fairness and justice, and do what is right even at times at a cost to themselves." The site offers parenting materials. https://mcc.gse.harvard.edu

CHAPTER 24

People Thrive When They Know They Matter

We humans thrive when we know we matter. Knowing we matter to others tells us we fit somewhere in the world and solidifies our sense of belonging. Knowing we matter drives our sense of purpose to make a difference to and for those around us. It strengthens our resolve to give to others in their times of need and hopefully allows us to draw from others' support more easily when we need it.

Knowing you matter is the foundational element of human resilience and thriving. It is laid in childhood and influenced most by parents. From the moment you attended to your baby's needs, they learned that they mattered to you. As your child grew and you celebrated their uniqueness, they experienced what it meant to be loved and began to understand their worth. Launching from the security of this knowledge, they become ready to matter to others, both in large and small ways.

Preparing for Adolescence

Adolescents receive an intense amount of pressure from many directions about "finding their purpose." If your child learns that they matter in ways large and small to people around them, when they reach adolescence, they'll feel a sense of belonging for being just who they are. They'll still want to do meaningful things but will do so out of a desire to make a difference rather than in response to pressures to perform.

Shaping Your Lifelong Bond

We do not need to change the world to know that we matter. We only need to be there for the person next to us. If your child, of any age, learns that they matter to another person, they will understand the vital lesson that their support and presence will always matter to you. This will pay off for decades to come as you continue to matter to each other.

The Roots of Mattering

To loved ones, you are valued

Your child will be "one of many" in every step along their lifelong journey—their school and playing fields now and in the work world in years to come. But in your home, they are truly unique. Therefore, your home is the place they can best be seen and valued and learn to value themselves. Let them see you enjoy them; they should know that their presence enriches your life! Ideally, your child will benefit from other people who love them: the other parent(s), extended family, the unconditional love of grandparents for those children lucky enough to have them in their lives. The bottom line is a child who knows they are valued by their loved ones—knows they matter.

To the community, you add value

Ultimately your child will draw their sense of mattering largely in their community, and when they are older, in the workplace. You prepare your child to know how much they matter outside of the home by practicing first within the home. Their home is the place to learn that they add value to others. Chores teach this lesson by creating experiences for children where they learn how they are a part of a "community" function. A small child can start simply by putting their toys back in the box. Older children can help with cooking, cleaning, home repairs, or taking care of younger children. It's never too early to allow children to contribute.

Our older children learn their value outside of our homes as well. They can choose to be helpful to an elderly neighbor. They can volunteer in the community to clean the environment, care for animals, or support those who are less fortunate. No matter your child's choice (emphasis on "their choice"), they will learn their presence adds value. That is a lifelong lesson.

A Note of Caution

Don't become a "cheerleader" that applauds every action your child takes or highlights every time they display good character. That can backfire for several reasons.

1. Your child needs to take your feedback seriously. If you praise every move they make—"Look at you being ready for school, you're so reliable!"—they won't listen as deeply when you're noticing and highlighting their most laudable character strengths such as generosity, integrity, and perseverance. Selective and deeply sincere feedback has more impact.

2. Many children feel they are always performing for the adults in their life. This generates pressure and leads to anxiety. Children should spend most of their time just being children. That makes it even more special when you notice the important and unique things they're doing.

3. As we discussed in Chapter 5, you want your child to know that it is the connection to you—your relationship—that matters most to you. If they believe they only get your attention when they're performing in ways that please you they may not come to you when they worry they'd displease you, and that is likely when they need you the most.

4. Children are uneven. People thrive when they're able to focus on developing their strengths and can recognize but not feel badly about their limitations. Focusing on your child's authentic strengths helps them to sharpen them. But if they feel as if everything they do is worthy of a cheer, it will undermine their ability to truly get to know themselves.

From Mattering to Meaning and Purpose

Finding our purpose unfolds over many years and is reinforced each time our presence matters. You cannot tell your child their purpose, but you can support them to find their own. You catalyze the pursuit of purpose when you encourage actions that will enable them to experience how much they matter to those around them. You reinforce the development of purpose when you notice and discuss the good you see your child doing.

A Sense of Purpose Holds Many Benefits

Research has demonstrated that people who feel a sense of purpose benefit in many ways, such as

- Having greater physical health and lower levels of stress hormones. This pays off in real ways that contribute to our well-being as we age. (Recall from Chapter 18 that the surgeon general reported the serious effects of loneliness. Knowing we matter to others may be a key motivation to choosing to remain connected.)
- Having a greater sense of satisfaction and happiness.
- Being driven by optimism and maintaining hope.
- Having increased resilience to navigate different environments or changing circumstances.
- Improved academic performance, including commitment to studying and completing homework.
- Better self-regulation.
- Improved perseverance and grit.

I strive to help parents, schools, and communities prepare young people to thrive. In one school setting, a psychologist and school counselor focused their attention on young people who had deep emotional distress and acted out in traditional school settings. They knew these students had the seeds of compassion within them but had not been able to break through their pervasive sense of hopelessness.

As a team, these mental health professionals took my teachings to heart that people who learn they matter to others might realize how much worth they possess. They invited these students to participate in volunteer projects around the school for an hour each week. The psychologist and counselor provided guidance, mentoring, and targeted feedback on the impact they made.

Over time, school staff and students noticed their contributions as well, giving them spontaneous positive feedback. Knowing they mattered instilled the self-worth in them that motivated them to reengage and succeed in school. At the end of this experience, one girl summarized, "I used to think I was going to die from what I was doing, and now I know I can change the world." If knowing they matter to others made such a difference to these teens' sense of purpose and reignited their motivation, imagine what it can do for your child.

We Don't Live on Posters

Take a moment to do a quick internet image search on the word "purpose." I'll bet you'll have 2 conflicting emotions as you scroll through the pictures: inspiration and intimidation. You may be inspired by people sitting on mountaintops after having climbed heights they'd never imagined. You may be moved by others gazing into sunsets, contemplating their role in improving the world. Perhaps you may also feel intimidated because you haven't scaled a mountain recently or arrived at a cogent plan to solve the world's challenges. The notion that pursuing a purpose must take you to such heights is more than intimidating; it might just shut down the pursuit of purpose.

If your child has not yet reached adolescence, it is challenging for them to authentically imagine themselves far into the future. Now is the time to lay the building blocks so they can develop into a human who ultimately may find a deeper sense of meaning and purpose in their lives. You do so by helping them understand how much they matter to those around them. If you have an adolescent, you might need to buffer them against the angst that "finding your purpose" can generate. "Finding your purpose" can contribute to magnifying stress in the high school years because it has been framed for too many students as a strategy to be accepted into top colleges. In turn, it's made too many high schoolers feel like failures because they haven't yet figured out how they are going to make their mark in the world, or feel like imposters because they pretend they have. People develop their purpose at their own pace, and expecting adolescents to solidify their life's purpose early on or even quickly is unfair and unrealistic. However, adolescence is about exploring one's identity, and finding how we fit into the world is an important part of that process. So, we *should* be supporting adolescents to imagine their purpose. But self-discovery is their work, and we must not rush them or inform them what we believe their purpose should be.

I believe deeply that our children are the leaders of tomorrow. And certainly, we need them to grow to build us a sustainable, just, and equitable world. I *do* believe in lofty goals. But we mustn't allow the pursuit of purpose to be framed only in the context of moving mountains lest we inadvertently exclude anyone from finding theirs. There is not a child or adolescent (or adult) on this planet who cannot learn that they live a purposeful life by being there for their family and friends. That should be the basis that we teach our children so that each of them can know that they matter. From the foundation of knowing that we matter to one another, people can confidently—and over time—develop a sense of meaning and purpose.

I have great respect for the work of Anthony Burrow, PhD, who directs the Purpose and Identity Processes Laboratory at Cornell University. He and his colleagues are ensuring that the conversation about purpose includes the fact that each of us can live a life of meaning. Rooted in an understanding that purpose is an important resource to enhance people's well-being, his team explores how we can give rise to a sense of purpose in adolescents. Among the areas he explores is the importance of *contribution*.

The beauty of contribution, also one of the 7 Cs discussed in Chapter 19, is that a child is never too young to learn that they contribute to others. Each of us contributes when we make our households function better. Each of us matters when we show up for another person in need. When we listen. When we respect. And when we care. If we take on this model of mattering, we all can learn how much our lives have a purpose.

A Parent's Supportive Role in Nurturing a Sense of Meaning and Purpose

Ultimately, your child's sense of purpose must arise from within them. You shouldn't say, "Your purpose is _____." Also, be careful not to apply indirect pressure by sharing what *you think* their purpose should be. Pressure of any kind, direct or indirect, can create internal conflict in children because they want to please you but also need to discover their own path. In the worst case, children may grow to resent positive actions if they feel forced or pressured to do them. This is a difficult balancing act to strike because sometimes we may see the strengths within our child, such as deep empathy, that they are not yet ready to see in themselves. Support your child in their journey of discovering their purpose without placing a timeline on their finding a purpose. Your role is to plant the seeds for your child to lead a purposeful life.

Members of the Adolescent Moral Development Lab at Claremont Graduate University, led by Kendall Cotton Bronk, PhD, summarized the science exploring the development of purpose and suggested 3 ways parents can help teens find their purpose. Although their focus was on adolescents, the lessons can be applied to children of an earlier age.

1. Help your child develop a sense of gratitude.
2. Expose your child to people who live a life of purpose and situations where they might discover how they matter.
3. Talk with your child about the things that matter to them to begin conversations about what they hope to accomplish.

Your child benefits by experiencing gratitude

Experiencing gratitude helps children feel satisfied with their own lives and better appreciate others. It also has been shown to improve mental health, perhaps partly because it increases connection to others. As children reflect on their own good fortunes, they may want to pay forward their own blessings and give to others, thereby becoming involved with others in a productive and meaningful manner. Strategies to help your child experience gratitude are discussed in greater detail in Chapter 26.

Expose your child to purposeful people and activities

When children experience how people make a difference in others' lives, they can imagine how they, too, might contribute. They learn this from watching you, witnessing how other adults (and children and teens!) matter, and learning through their own experiences how much they can make a difference.

Discuss *why* you do what you do. Discuss how contributing to others brings meaning to your life. "I volunteer at the food bank because I believe hunger shouldn't exist in our nation." Or, "When I was growing up, a teacher guided me on how to reach my potential, so I decided I would be there for kids and make sure every young person believes in themselves." As you model how your purpose enriches you, share those moments where knowing you mattered gave you the strength to overcome challenges in your own life.

Encourage your child to step outside their comfort zone. We want our children to know that many people do not have enough and that we as humans must course correct some actions to maintain the health of the planet. It is important, however, to not expose your child to more than they can process, and this is related to their developmental stage. So, if you're watching a documentary or witnessing inequities, do it alongside your child so you can gauge what they understand and answer their questions. Don't force them to try to grasp what they might not be ready to see.

Encourage volunteer work. As your child gets older, they can find time to give service. They may find satisfaction in these volunteer activities, largely because volunteer activities offer powerful opportunities for each of us to experience how much we can matter. Volunteering doesn't always mean working on an official project or within an agency; it can also mean simply offering the most precious gift—time—to someone who will benefit from their presence. Even 8- or 9-year-olds can help a neighbor who is homebound complete chores. Sometimes the greatest gift a child can give is their joyful presence. Your child might choose to spend time with an elderly or disabled person, just offering them some company. In so doing, they will likely hear stories and learn from their neighbor's wisdom and experience. Giving service to others is a win-win for all involved.

Talk With Your Child About Their Strengths

Every child possesses unique strengths, talents, and potential. If your child is older, you might explicitly discuss how these strengths might flavor what they hope to accomplish in the world. If your child is a pre-tween, help them reflect on how their strengths make them the kind of person who can brighten other lives, today and every day.

Resources

"The Psychology of Purpose" is a comprehensive assessment of the science of purpose. It was created by the members of the Adolescent Moral Development Lab at Claremont Graduate University for Prosocial Consulting and the John Templeton Foundation. It is accessible at https://www.templeton.org/wp-content/uploads/2020/02/Psychology-of-Purpose.pdf.
VolunteerMatch matches people with opportunities to contribute to their communities, connecting volunteers with nonprofits. https://www.volunteermatch.org

CHAPTER 25

People Who Thrive: Curiosity and a Growth Mindset Are Key

You do not need to develop a love of learning in your child; it is already there! The drive to explore the world and satisfy curiosity is a gift that comes with childhood. Your job is to encourage your child to understand that each experience and exposure is an opportunity for growth and to protect them from forces that might extinguish their natural curiosity.

Curiosity is about wanting to know more. It drives us to uncover meaningful answers and therefore can lead to a greater sense of purpose. It also leads us to seek wisdom from people with different life experiences. In turn, this encourages a collaborative nature because as curiosity drives us to better understand others' points of view, it encourages us to incorporate their wisdom as we problem-solve. Curiosity also brings joy. It allows us to see the *extra*ordinary within the ordinary and to experience wonder in our everyday lives.

Preparing for Adolescence

Adolescence is the second phase of "whys." Adolescents are as curious as toddlers, but they want to explore deeper topics. They want to know how things *really* work. Raising a child who has a growth mindset ensures their natural curiosity will lead them to success during the teen years.

Shaping Your Lifelong Bond

People should never lose their love of learning. When your adult child sees you as the person who encouraged them to savor life and stretch into new territories, they may forever see you as someone they want by their side to seek out new adventures.

Your Role in Fostering Your Child's Curiosity

According to Susan Engel, PhD, senior lecturer in psychology at Williams College, 3- to 4-year-olds ask a question a minute! That is exhilarating, even if it is exhausting to be on the receiving end. Dr Engel has written 2 important books, *The Hungry Mind: The Origins of Curiosity in Childhood* and *The Intellectual Lives of Children*. One of the key points she makes is that studies of curiosity prove what you likely already know. *Children who ask a lot of questions and receive satisfying answers grow to wisely continue to ask more questions.* You likely took so much pride in your child's curiosity and responded to their endless questions partly because you knew it was a sign of their growing intelligence and was their path to gain confidence to explore the world. Don't stop now! Families where questions are encouraged raise children who know their curiosity is valued.

To elevate curiosity in your child, first just choose to not extinguish the innate wonder of childhood. We know that as children grow they may start to ask fewer questions; aim to be the kind of parent who raises a human whose curiosity is never diminished. To toddlers and young children, the world is designed for discovery. As they grow, they might spend so much time trying to be more grown up (and forgetting to play!) that they miss the miracles they walk past every day. Science is not just in books; it is everywhere, as is poetry. Once again, I'm going to highlight how critical you, the parent, are as a role model.

Slow down and notice the mysteries that surround you. Blow more bubbles and wonder how the rainbows are created within them. Let the child within you out, the one filled with curiosity and joy. Your child will see this and benefit, but maybe not as much as you will.

The bottom line is a curious person understands that the world holds unlimited opportunities to learn and to expand our existing understanding. The following are some thoughts to foster your child's innate curiosity:

Notice curiosity. If your child asks a question that gets you excited, tell them! Let them know how pleased you are that their questions help you grow too.

Say "I don't know" when you don't know. If you know or pretend to know all the answers, children may feel frustrated when they don't know something. Instead, we want them to be curious enough to search for answers.

Follow "I don't know" with, "But I'm going to find out!" Model how your curiosity drives your growth. Help your child see that when you aren't sure about something you'll seek answers, and that it's OK to do so.

Share your excitement. If you're interested in something, show it! Model how you follow your interests to learn more.

Be an explorer. Children who ask a lot of questions tend to have curious parents. When your child has a question you can't answer *yet*, come together as a team of explorers, or engage them to explore on their own.

Ask open-ended questions that seek deeper explanations. When you are the one asking the questions, avoid asking questions that can be answered with a simple "yes" or "no" because those monosyllabic answers stop exploration. Learn to ask "how" and "why" questions and then encourage your child to explain their discoveries to you.

Provide meaningful answers to questions (or find someone who can). Your child will ask deeper questions when they receive interesting answers. Again, don't feel like you're supposed to have all the answers. Just encourage your child to continue to seek out those answers. Let them know that there are many people—besides you—who might have the answers. This will encourage both exploration and collaboration.

Create good mysteries. Everyone wants to solve a mystery. Imagine together what the answer might be. Take a good guess! Then encourage your child to solve the mystery.

End your days with a family share session. At the end of each day, gather your family together for a few moments to share something each person learned. Even better if people talk about something that piqued their interest but they haven't *yet* learned. Everyone will look forward to the future discussion that reveals the lesson learned!

The Mindset for Success

To guide our children toward success, we should foster a growth mindset. This allows them to be self-reflective and to be comfortable with their strengths and limitations. You start this by valuing your child's curiosity. A curious person is excited to venture into new territory and knows each misstep is an opportunity to learn.

This discussion is deeply influenced by the work of Carol Dweck, PhD, a Stanford University psychologist whose decades of research guides us on how to hold young people to high expectations in a way that fosters, rather than undermines their performance, while also attending to their emotional well-being. Her book, *Mindset: The New Psychology of Success*, may shift how you approach raising your child as you apply practical strategies on how to optimize performance and well-being in childhood and adolescence. You will likely find pearls within her work that will help you build your own growth mindset in ways that may help you both personally and within the workplace. Critically, your own growth mindset will position you to better support your child to develop their own.

Growth versus fixed mindset

Intelligence has been (wrongly) measured in a way that presumes it is fixed—something that will not change. Dr Dweck and many others have proven intelligence can be built through exposure, exploration, and experience. Children (and adults!) with a growth mindset are willing to put in the effort to develop their intelligence. They know that stretching will expose them to their existing limitations; they learn to not see themselves as failures when they make a mistake but as learners who can surmount setbacks. They seek constructive feedback so they can learn how to improve. And the ability to respond to constructive feedback is undoubtedly linked with academic and workplace success. Dr Dweck summarizes, "The passion for stretching yourself and sticking to it even (or especially) when it's not going well is the hallmark of the growth mindset."

People with a fixed mindset may experience failure and view it as proof that they are not smart and feel like impostors and undeserving even when they succeed. They may avoid tasks that require hard work for fear of it signaling to others, or reinforcing within themselves, that the task did not come naturally to them. They may not venture outside the box, where real innovations exist, because they fear failure or even setbacks. They may view feedback as criticism and therefore avoid it at all costs, stifling their growth. Can you see how all of this interferes with the love of learning or may even extinguish curiosity?

People with a growth mindset seek expanded horizons while those with fixed mindsets feel wise when they stay within safe and familiar territory. You want your child to feel joy as they stretch because their growth mindset will produce academic successes and interpersonal gains as they more comfortably meet people with diverse life experiences and lead them to enriching experiences throughout life.

How praise can support a growth mindset

We convey our high expectations when we notice our children's actions, praise their best efforts, and offer gentle criticism when they go astray. To support a growth mindset in your child, you might need to unlearn some of what you have been taught about fostering their self-esteem. A generation of parents and educators were taught that effusive praise made a child feel good about themselves. Each child was reassured they were as "special as a butterfly" and "unique as a snowflake." We cheered as children came down the park slide, raved about their bravery, and treated the accomplishment as theirs alone. We never suggested gravity was on their side.

We *should* notice and cheer children's accomplishments, but overpraising backfires for several reasons. First, effusive and general praise misses the opportunity to offer the kind of targeted praise that reinforces specific accomplishments and guides children on which actions they should repeat. Second, effusive praise that makes children feel good all the time misses the opportunity to prepare them for challenging moments when they won't feel like the center of attention. Third, when our eyes are on our children's every action, it can make them feel as though they are performing for us rather than living their lives. Fourth, effusive, untargeted praise highlights a child's attributes—smart, talented, brave—but misses the opportunity to reinforce the actions they did to arrive there—studying, practicing, and/or finding their inner strength.

Dr Dweck teaches that words of praise can send a message about how children should think about themselves. Consider comments like, "You are so smart! You are such a great player/performer/artist!" Are we communicating that they have a fixed trait such as intelligence or talent? When we emphasize what they *are*, children may feel judged and are more likely to think their current state is permanent and defines them. This may generate fear of failure because they worry about losing their status. Communicate instead that you see your child as a developing person, capable of growth, and poised to learn from each new experience.

To build your child's authentic self-confidence and genuine self-esteem, shift your feedback from, "You are _____," to, "You did _____ and therefore, _____ happened." For example, rather than saying, "You are so good at math and that test proved it!" say, "You studied hard, completed your homework, and asked for help when you needed it. You were prepared for the test and it paid off." When a child knows they accomplished a task because of what they did, they'll feel empowered with the knowledge of how to continue to build on their successes.

How criticism can support a growth mindset

Criticism wisely offered in the spirit of self-improvement can support a growth mindset. Here are 3 basic points.

1. Criticism must be specific to an action. It should never focus on something your child can't change.
2. Constructive criticism should use your child's existing strengths as starting points to improvement.
3. Criticism should always offer a path toward improvement.

Criticism must never sound like, "You are _____," which suggests you're commenting on a fixed trait. You don't want your child to react to your feedback with an internal dialogue such as, "Well, if I am _____, I can't change, so I won't even try." If, on the other hand, when you say, "You did _____," your child knows they controlled what happened. Now put this together with strength-based communication. "You did _____ and this is not the behavior I like to see. I know you can do better because you do _____ so often."

Let's consider an example. Sonia didn't help her mother prepare her little sister for her second-grade play. If her mother says, "You always think of yourself, and you let your sister down," Sonia feels ashamed and begins to see herself as self-centered. She perceives that her family expects her to be unhelpful. Frustrated and feeling she has nothing to lose, she may refuse to help in the future. Imagine if her mother had said, "You didn't come through for your sister when she needed your help. This isn't like you because you are so loving toward her. That's why you are her hero. Next time, I need you to plan your day so you have time to help out when we need you. Now let's go to the play and show her how proud we are!" Through this communication, Sonia knows what is expected of her, has a suggestion on how to improve, and will hopefully rise to that expectation next time. And the family has a night where they can celebrate the joy of watching her sister's theatrical debut!

Cautionary note: Never offer criticism when angry. Angry words are driven by rage or disappointment. You don't want to make the mistake of suggesting your child really is how they behave at their worst. When calm, you'll focus on their strengths and root your feedback in the belief that they can do better.

Refer to the following tables for suggestions of what to say and avoid saying when offering praise or criticism. The examples underscore 3 key points.

- Praise effort rather than outcome to reinforce that your child has control.
- Notice actions (what was done) rather than the result.
- Be specific and targeted with either praise or criticism, rather than making a general statement.

Praise

Say This	Not That
What did you learn in school today?	Did you get a good grade on the test?
Is the coach helping your team learn how to communicate on the field better?	How many goals did you score?
Were you proud of your display in the science exhibition?	Did you win the top prize?
I appreciate how you're always asking questions to learn more.	You're so smart.
Tell me about your picture. It captures so many feelings.	You're a great artist.
You did well on your math test because you did all of your homework and asked your big brother to help you with the problems you didn't yet understand. You refused to give up!	Math comes naturally to you.
I really respect how you're not afraid to ask for help. Did you see how it paid off because you learned how to do something you were struggling with?	See how good you are at this! You didn't believe you could do it!

Criticism

Say This	Not That
You didn't study and you weren't prepared. You spent last night focused on social media instead of with your books.	You don't care about learning. That's why you're getting bad grades.
You are distracted. Step away for a few minutes to regain your focus.	The way you are staring into space makes me feel like you just don't care about the game.
Why do you think your grades dropped on this last test?	If you're this lazy, your grades will continue to disappoint us.
I was counting on you to watch your sisters after school. When I learned you were on the other side of town without a ride, I had to change my meetings. You need to learn to better keep track of your commitments.	You are so irresponsible. Maybe just once, you could realize how much I do for you and step up to help around here.
Your cousin needed your help tonight, but you didn't show up for him. He looks up to you and is so appreciative when you help him with homework.	You went out with your friends and completely forgot about your cousin. You can be so self-centered.

Failure: The First Step Toward Meaningful Growth

Too many people believe that if they experience failure, they *are* a failure. This is partly because the word "failure" itself sounds so permanent and feels like a label. We must learn to see failure as a *temporary* state that offers an opportunity for growth. Failure can feel awful in the moment but *always* offers the kind of lesson that allows us to grow.

It's natural for parents to want to protect their children from discomfort. But if you prevent mistakes they can grow from now, they'll experience more failures later that may lead to much greater consequences. Childhood and adolescence are the time to learn those "workarounds" for our limitations that we'll need throughout life. These strategies to compensate for our weaknesses allow us to sharpen our strengths because we'll have fewer failures to consume our energy.

The need to learn how to recover from failure is critical to learning to succeed. Why? Because we can build on our strengths. Our greatest successes come over time after multiple attempts and continued improvements. But if we stay in safe and comfortable territory, we'll remain just that—comfortable. We won't generate new ideas or reach our potential. Each misstep generates new knowledge. When we stretch and "fail" it is because we are venturing out of our safe zones. Our progress, and ultimately success, relies on experimentation and growth from each misstep.

Your child needs to learn that mistakes lead to growth, not to catastrophes. (See Chapter 21 for a discussion on catastrophic thinking.) When they grasp this, they'll learn to work with their imperfections and be guided by their strengths to stretch into new territory. I'm not suggesting that you should push your child to choose to fail. But I am saying that when they experience life's inevitable failures and learn that you stand beside them and encourage them to learn life's lessons, they'll more comfortably seek growth opportunities.

CHAPTER 26

Living With Gratitude and a Generous Spirit Is Core to Thriving

We want our children to know that they deserve to be loved, to be showered with attention, and to never lack the necessities of life. We hope they embrace the comforts and joys that enrich life and the opportunities that open their eyes to new experiences. But we *also* want them to count their blessings rather than assume they are entitled to all they desire. This sense of appreciation, or gratitude, will allow them to walk more humbly through life because they realize their good fortunes and understand they need to continue to earn them.

Experiencing gratitude is linked to developing a generous spirit. An authentically appreciative child begins to grasp that the giver was intentional about their action and themselves felt rewarded by their generosity. This is true whether the act of generosity was a material gift like a toy that makes a child beam ear to ear or a sweater that offers comfort and warmth, or the greatest gift of all, time and nurturance. When your child realizes that humans who give generously are enriched themselves, they learn the vital lesson that their own generosity will connect them to others in meaningful ways.

To those to whom much is given, much is expected. We will build a better world when our children want to pay their blessings forward and enrich the lives of others.

Preparing for Adolescence

If you raise your child to feel authentically grateful for what they have, they will have greater appreciation about how life really works and will be better prepared to thrive on their own. You also might find they'll appreciate you more because they've thoughtfully considered the intention and effort it takes to meet their basic and emotional needs.

Shaping Your Lifelong Bond

You hope to share your life with your adult child for decades to come. "Share" is the key word here. That means you will give and receive. I'm not speaking here of objects or possessions but of the things we should be most grateful for—unconditional love, sage advice, meaningful experiences, and generosity of spirit. Focus on helping your child know these are the things to be truly grateful for and you'll raise an adult who will know how much you matter to each other.

Please and Thank You

Do you remember the first time your child expressed gratitude? It may not have felt as life-changing as their first steps (because you quickly had to learn to scurry after them!) but it was a momentous milestone, nonetheless. It was the first step in your child learning that their needs are not magically met.

One of my most cherished memories is the too-big-for-their-little-hands "please-thank-you-please-thank you" apple. At the time, my 20-month-old girls stood next to each other and chortled with glee as they passed a shiny red apple back and forth, squeaking "please" as they asked for their turn and "thank you" after they received the apple. It took their tiny little teeth at least 100 back-and- forths to make a serious dent in their shared treasure. I looked on with pride and belly laughed as I watched these 2 little beings mimic the words they must have heard us model.

The First Step Is Being Appreciated

We want our children to be polite because we know having manners allows them to present themselves in a positive light. But it is authentic gratitude, really meaning it, that offers the richer emotional experience that connects us to others.

The first step to your child appreciating others is for them to learn firsthand how good it feels to be appreciated themselves. Your child is never too young to contribute to your household. When they make their contribution, let them know that you appreciate them going out of their way to be helpful. This includes any chores that you've set for them, but make sure to especially notice the special efforts they choose to be helpful. If you do, I'll bet you'll see your child being helpful more often. More importantly, notice and reinforce through your appreciation their displays of empathy and kindness. When they support another person, highlight how thoughtful they are being. This will instill in them an understanding that the time we make for others takes intention and thoughtfulness.

Be Mindful of Good Things

Most of us spend a lot of time focusing on our problems, worries, or to-do lists. The clichéd phrase, "Don't forget to smell the flowers," reminds us to notice and appreciate the little things. National holidays such as Veteran's Day and Martin Luther King Day instill a sense of appreciation for those who have sacrificed for us. But phrases and holidays alone don't give us the push to move past our worries and experience all we should be grateful for.

We spend so much time focusing on our worries because many of the gifts we experience have become routine. You know what might serve as an ongoing reminder of all you are grateful for? A young person like your child. If we love what we do at work, sometimes it takes the fresh eyes of the person in training to remind us how lucky we are to do what we do. To our children, so much is new. When we spend time with them, we are reminded of how much we might take for granted because so much seems fresh and interesting to them. As they remind us to be grateful, they learn through our renewed excitement to continue to appreciate even the routine in their lives.

How *Not* to Instill Gratitude

Guilt. Don't use it. I assure you that reminding your child how deserving you are of their gratitude will not make them appreciate you more. So don't start your days with, "Do you know I could've slept in but instead I cooked breakfast for you and now all you're doing is staring into your phone?" That will only drive them to prefer cold cereal. Don't end your days either with, "I am exhausted after a long day's work, and I can't imagine adding one more thing to my plate. But you're worth it, and I'm happy to help." Children don't want to feel as if you're sacrificing for them. It will only push them into feeling guilty and asking for less. In this case, it may prevent them from asking for homework support.

I also didn't mean to instill guilt in you either. I am *not* suggesting you are supposed to experience nothing but pleasure as you give to your children. You are human! You deserve downtime as much as they do. I expect you will have many moments when there is no part of you that wants to give, give, give, and instead wants to scream that it's your turn to receive or at least do nothing. I caution you, however, to be careful about what feelings you convey to your child. This is yet another example where self-care benefits you both. Fill your cup and let others be generous with you at times. You deserve nothing less. Once you feel cared for, it will be far easier to give to your child.

Notice, Think, Feel, Do

Dr Andrea Hussong, professor of psychology and neuroscience at the University of North Carolina, has explored how to instill genuine gratitude in our children. First, she emphasizes that it is a developmental process and that children of different ages have varying abilities to fully experience gratitude. Our goal as parents is to help them build a deeper sense of gratitude over time in the hope they will grow to fully experience its benefits.

She proposed the notice, think, feel, do model. The last step, do, is likely the first step your children will take and is the one parents are most likely to reinforce. "Say thank you." "Did you call your grandma to let her know how much you liked the cookies she sent?" The dos are easy for us to notice. But even in the "do" category we can broaden our children's understanding of gratitude. It's easy for them to recognize the material gifts that require our gratitude. Help your child understand that time generously given also merits appreciation. After all, time being genuinely listened to is an authentic gift. Another example is the playful attention an adult gives a child because the adult chooses to spend time in a way that allows the child to set the rules and explain their world.

We can support our children in having a richer experience with gratitude when we activate their thinking and feelings. The first step of thinking is noticing. Life gives us many opportunities to be grateful. Some are visible, like gifts. These generate the easiest dos. Some we too often take for granted—nourishment, shelter, clothing. Some enrich our experience of living, but we are too caught up in the hustle of the day to offer them our attention and focused appreciation—flowers, sunsets. And others give our life meaning, pleasure, and security, like love and friendships.

We should take the moments to stop and notice things too easily passed by, and then describe to our children what we notice. "Let's pull over to the side of the road and watch the sun go down." You can also ask your child specific questions like, "What happened today that you really appreciated?" Consider rituals that force your family to slow down, take notice, and appreciate what we're given. Sharing blessings or saying grace before eating is a ritual that makes eating an intentional act and reminds people that good food should not be taken for granted.

We make meaning out of what we notice by using our thoughts and feelings. We can do this when we discuss with our children the "whys" that explain what they have received. This helps them grasp how much thought others placed on their material gifts or their time and attention. "Why do you think Grandpa baked you that cake?" A younger child might say, "Because it tastes good." A child further in development will appreciate the real intention behind the act, "Because he was thinking of me and wants to make me happy." "Why do you think your friend's mother welcomes you to their home after school and has a snack ready for you?" A younger child might say, "Well, she's here anyway." The older child who's developing a deeper sense of gratitude might say, "Because you are still at work, and she likes making sure we're both safe."

When we help our children experience gratitude on the feeling level, it can add a deeper understanding of gratitude. "Now that you understand Grandpa made that treat because he loves you, how does that make you feel?" "How does it make you feel to know that Ms_____ is going out of her way to welcome you into her home?" When your child begins to realize that others' actions bring them happiness and security, their gratitude grows, and we hope their desire to do for others is nurtured. After all, they'll want to pass along good feelings to others.

It is not surprising that research has demonstrated that most parents focus on what their children are doing to express gratitude (politeness, writing "old-fashioned" thank-you notes). After all, this is what we notice, can verify, and can reinforce (or force!). But since these actions may not represent the best way for your child to develop authentic gratitude, we want to broaden how our children *react* to physical gifts or the gift of time, intention, and love. Let's think about things we might do or say in each category to broaden our children's experiences.

In the following table, we'll look at different experiences of how you can deepen the understanding and appreciation of gratitude. Saying *why* the experience is meaningful underscores your child's ability to think about something they should be grateful for. It makes our thoughts and feelings visible to our children. Our discussion helps all of us—adults and children—feel gratitude. Ultimately, as in every aspect of parenting, when we model the full experience, our children learn the most. Especially in something where richness develops over time, like gratitude, modeling demonstrates what brings meaning to our lives.

Notice It	Say It	Discuss It	Model It
Take a moment to notice your meal rather than just starting to eat. For families that say grace or words of thanks, there is an intentional pause before eating.	"I am fortunate to be able to share this wonderful dinner with my family. We're lucky to have nourishing food and to be able to spend time together."	"It's easy to go through life and not count our blessings. Do you ever think about how many people were involved in bringing this meal together? The farmer, the grocer. Even me as the chef and you as the cleaner-upper."	If you truly feel fortunate, savor what you are given. Enjoy the food rather than rush through it. Take advantage of the time you are given together. Tip: Ensure cell phones are off. Share your time fully present.
When receiving a gift, notice the thought that went behind it.	"Your aunt put so much thought into your present. She knows how creative you are and gave you something so you can continue to express yourself."	"I love the picture you painted. The colors draw me in, and I can almost hear the birds chirping in your picture."	"I'm going to send your aunt a picture of your painting. She deserves to know that her thoughtfulness has given you an opportunity to continue to build your creative side."
When your neighbor comes to watch your children so you can go out, take a pause to genuinely reflect that someone is giving you the gift of time.	"I am going to enjoy being out tonight. It will be even better because I know you're going to be watched by someone who really cares about you."	"Mrs _____ is giving this family the greatest gift of all, which is time and attention to recharge. She enjoys you so much that she's giving up her own time so we can go out."	"I'm going to have the neighbors' children join us on Saturday. We're going to have a fun movie and popcorn night. I'm also doing it so their parents will have some special time together."

Gratitude Leads to Generosity

When we experience gratitude, it fuels our drive to give to others. The connection between gratitude and generosity is precisely what builds stronger families and, indeed, communities. Giving to one another builds cohesive communities in which we can all thrive.

There is a deep root of human generosity that reveals itself even in toddlers. Think back to your own young child, and I'll bet you can recall them demonstrating generosity as toddlers. In fact, Dr Julia Ulber and her colleagues at the Department of Developmental and Comparative Psychology, Max Planck Institute for Evolutionary Anthropology, found that pairs of 18- to 24-month-olds divided small treasures (OK, it was marbles) even when one had to sacrifice some of their own to ensure equality. So, the desire to be generous and consider someone else's needs seems to be innately wired into us. Yet, selfish desires are also wired into us, and I'm not suggesting that you raise your child to be entirely selfless. Rather, I am stating that we all thrive when our culture encourages us to have a generous spirit, one that inspires us to care for others.

The Greater Good Science Center prepared a report for the John Templeton Foundation in 2018 called *The Science of Generosity*. I don't think it will surprise you to learn that it described many benefits to the giver. It revealed that generosity was associated with better overall health in older adults and volunteering was associated with longer life. Generosity is linked to psychological health and well-being. It has even been linked to feeling greater vitality and self-esteem. All of this leads to happiness. Generous people benefit in the workplace, where they have a reduced likelihood of burnout. Finally, but perhaps most telling, generous people feel more contentment in their romantic relationships, and those relationships tend to last longer.

Knowing this, let's consider 5 things you can do to nurture your child's generosity.

1. **Build your child's sense of gratitude.** This is a freebie because applying everything we've discussed in this chapter will contribute to you raising a generous child.
2. **Model generosity in your own life.** Discuss why you choose to give to others. Is it out of a sense of fairness? Of sharing joy? Of wanting others to feel cared about?
3. **Uncover passion areas.** Search for opportunities that allow your child to share their interests. Are they passionate about animals? They can volunteer their time at the local pet rescue. Young people are more likely to give generously when they care about the cause.
4. **Help them reflect on their experiences being on the receiving end.** When they grasp how good it feels to receive, especially when they focus

on the whys, they'll want to learn for themselves how good it can feel to give to others.

5. **Promote humility.** Humble people appreciate how much others can contribute to the world. These people are also more generous. Humility prevents judgment, and judgment gets in the way of us wanting to support others.

The generosity of forgiveness

One of the most generous things we can do for another person is to be forgiving of them when they are not their best selves. As we discussed in Chapter 5, when we are forgiving of ourselves it reassures our children that we will be forgiving of them when they need it, and that makes them more likely to come to us when they need us the most. Modeling forgiveness in your home is also critical to allowing us to move forward, repair relationships, and even grow together. This will be discussed further in Chapter 31. For now, know that "I'm sorry" goes a long way in helping when any of us—parent or child—hurts one another through a mistake in behavior or a missed opportunity to offer needed support.

The lesson of forgiveness may be genuinely driven home best by asking for forgiveness for our own human lapses and mistakes. A genuine apology states that a lesson has been learned. "I am so sorry that my frustration from work made me seem angry with you when all you wanted was for me to spend time with you. I didn't just promise you that time, I cherish that time with you. I let you down and made you feel bad. Forgive me? Can you make time with me now? I've had my cool-off time and talked out my feelings. I feel so much better."

What Goes Around Comes Around

As your child learns to experience gratitude more fully, you may find them being more generous with you. The key is for them to better understand how intentional people (including you) are with the time and attention they offer. Equipped with the understanding of how genuinely thoughtful you are with them, they may have the desire to communicate how much they appreciate you. It'll start out with objects such as the pictures that adorn your refrigerator. Hopefully, as your child grows, they will understand that offering time, support, nurturance, and forgiveness are immeasurably important ways we display generosity with one another.

CHAPTER 27

We Thrive When We Remain Open to Learning From Others

Being open to others' thoughts and feelings does not diminish or deny our own. When we approach the world with a growth mindset, as discussed in Chapter 25, we can amplify our knowledge, sharpen our thoughts, and feel our feelings more fully, precisely because we have been exposed to new ideas and perspectives. In fact, admitting what we don't know *yet* doesn't imply a deficit of intelligence but, rather, reveals an openness to growth.

A healthy society relies on respectful discussion between people of varied views to arrive at the best strategies to meet the needs of its citizenry. But many people stoke division for personal gain and promote an "us versus them" mindset that suggests that the only way to achieve gains is to ensure "the other side" somehow loses. I am deeply worried about this on 2 levels. First, as a citizen of a great nation I worry that our potential is being squandered. Second, as a child and adolescent advocate, I am concerned that our children are absorbing the tension between adults and being made to feel less secure in the present, fearful of the future, and less hopeful about the power of civic engagement. And if this generation of children and teens are dissuaded from becoming involved in solution-building efforts, both on local and national levels, because of adult leaders behaving badly and irresponsibly today, I mourn for the lost potential leadership of tomorrow.

We can nurture our children to be open to learning from others. We want them to learn to think for themselves and to have confidence in their own ideas. But we want them also to know that their own knowledge, wisdom, and experience has limitations. When we remain respectful and receptive to others' existing knowledge, earned wisdom, and gained experience we narrow our own limitations. This is what it means to be intellectually humble.

Preparing for Adolescence

Humility is about listening well and respectfully. You want your adolescent to develop their own thoughts, feelings, and opinions while also respecting yours. Undoubtedly, they will more likely remain open to your wisdom and guidance if you are open to learning from them and are receptive to their growing wisdom.

Shaping Your Lifelong Bond

Nobody wants to have a close relationship with another person who doesn't value their views. When you are respectful of your child's views and avoid telling them how you think they *should* think, your adult child will remain open to your wisdom far into the future. Your respect for their thoughts, which may vary from your own, is the root of their developing the intellectual humility that allows them to learn from others, including you, far into the future.

A Love of Learning

A love of learning helps humans thrive and deepens our emotional connections. I was raised to believe a person who loves learning could live a happy life while growing through every life experience. My relatives discussed this in my presence for a reason. They spoke of their voracious appetite for new knowledge and discussed the adult learning opportunities they engaged with in community and cultural centers. These open-minded relatives also took pride in their ability to think for themselves. They used their well-formed opinions to have (respectful but heated) discussions. Even when expressing themselves strongly, they never stopped listening to others and being enriched by their varied views. In the moments when they discussed big questions and the solutions they sought, they'd pass along well-earned cultural wisdom: "Knowledge is something you own that can never be taken from you. Think for yourself, but always be willing and ready to learn from others. Otherwise, how can you trust that you really know what is best?"

Intellectual humility

A humble person may have a great deal to share, but they value listening as much as they do talking. They grasp that wisdom is often earned from life experiences and respect those with firsthand knowledge. They honor the wisdom of years and thus hold the elderly in high esteem. They know that the unvarnished wisdom in children reminds us that curiosity is the greatest driver of knowledge.

Being humble doesn't mean you must deny your expertise. In fact, a person with well-earned know-how would do a disservice to those who might benefit from their expertise or experience if they were falsely humble. When they teach others how to rise closer to their level of expertise, they make an invaluable contribution. An expert remains humble when they understand that no matter how much they know they could always learn more from someone with a different perspective. On the other hand, such a person would be arrogant if they refused to share their knowledge, belittled others who had not yet acquired their knowledge, or thought they had little left to learn.

Dr Mark Leary, professor emeritus of psychology and neuroscience at Duke University, summarized key findings on intellectual humility for the John Templeton Foundation. He describes intellectual humility as ". . . a mindset that guides our intellectual conduct. In particular, it involves recognizing and owning our intellectual limitations in the service of pursuing deeper knowledge, truth, and understanding." He explains it is critical to good citizenship because "It promises to help us avoid headstrong decisions and erroneous opinions and allows us to engage more constructively with our fellow citizens."

People with intellectual humility tend to be more tolerant of differing views and are less likely to be condescending to those with whom they disagree. They are more likely to find common ground and less likely to get into heated arguments. This does not mean they don't hold well-thought-out opinions but, rather, that they remain open-minded with an eye toward growth. They avidly listen and therefore are better positioned to collaborate with and thereby influence others.

Do you see how intellectual humility might be connected to success? If you want to raise your child prepared for success, continued growth, and deep connection to others, this is an incredibly important character strength to reinforce!

Your role in encouraging intellectual humility

When you notice your child setting aside their own needs to honor those of others or being flexible in their thinking as they consider another child's perspective, let them know how much they have pleased you. Our children, no matter their age, want to make us proud. In many cases, simply noticing those demonstrations of humility and offering an approving look will be enough reinforcement. But occasionally, discuss how much you appreciate their openness to others' thoughts, feelings, and perspectives. Underscore how much those behaviors please you both because they demonstrate your child's essential goodness and also because this openness will be a key to their own success and well-being.

Flexibility and openness are virtues. However, it is also virtuous to maintain your own values with issues that involve safety, morality, or a commitment to justice. And it remains important to advocate for your own needs, not in a way that is selfish but in a way that allows you to thrive. We want our children to know that just as they learn from others, they can offer their own wisdom and experience in a way that can positively influence others. I say this clearly to ensure that while we raise our children to be intellectually humble, we also raise them to care for and about others and to advocate for their own needs.

Reinforce the seeds of humility

It might seem that with the word "intellectual" placed in front of humility, that this strength can be developed only once your child has developed their intellect. In fact, the seeds of intellectual humility are likely sown in the very early years. Sharing. Taking turns. Listening. Acknowledging others' needs. Learning that guidance from others is often protective. Each time you reinforce these seeds of humility, you raise your child to be open to others' perspectives and needs. Every step you take in building a growth mindset in your child by choosing how and when to appropriately praise and criticize lends itself to building the foundations of intellectual humility.

Model humility every day

Intellectual humility may be better modeled than taught. You are a model of the adult your child would like to be. Most of this modeling will come easily and will benefit you and your relationship with your child. Following are some ideas:

Be curious. The strategies described in Chapter 25 to encourage curiosity in your child will also foster their intellectual humility. Curious people know that exposure to others' ideas is an effective pathway toward new knowledge.

Remain open-minded and demonstrate flexibility. Our children watch our interactions and respect when we are willing to be open-minded. They even respect when they see our ability to learn from mistakes. Drive the lesson home by discussing when your viewpoints shifted because new (or better) information presented itself. You might say, "I used to think _____, but now I understand _____."

Seek knowledge. Start with what you know and be transparent about what you don't. Demonstrate that you seek information to learn more.

Know your biases. All people have biases. This does not make us bad; it makes us human. What makes us behave with humility is when we understand that we exist with biases and reflect on them and sometimes confront them before we make thoughtful decisions. You might say to your child, "Do you think you are making an assumption about that person that may not be fair? How can you find out what they really think?"

When your child makes you think differently, tell them! When we see the world through our children's eyes, we suddenly gain a new perspective. Our teen's idealism and commitment to building a better world can make you reconsider your own beliefs or opinions. Let your children know that their views can change yours. Seize the opportunity to say, "I've never thought of it like that, thank you!"

Model humility even when it may be hard

Dr Eranda Jayawickreme, from the Department of Psychology at Wake Forest University, studies intellectual humility and shared with the Center for Parent and Teen Communication strategies to encourage this critical character strength, especially in your interactions with others that may challenge your existing views or lead to disagreement.

- Adopt the viewpoint of someone impartially observing a situation, like a fly on the wall, rather than seeing it from your own perspective. This can help reduce the impact of biases we may have.
- We may disagree with another person's view. But we must resist seeing people we disagree with as inferior, less than, or as "others."
- When you are having a disagreement, frame it as an opportunity to learn about others and to benefit from their different outlook.
- Recognize the limits of your own knowledge. Understand that real intellectual growth comes by understanding that the more we learn, the more we understand that we have so much more to learn. This

understanding can fuel our growth and our desire to collaborate with others.

- Notice the feedback you receive. Ask yourself, "Are people unlikely to challenge me because of a position I may hold or power I may have in the relationship?" If you recognize that your position may prevent people from sharing their earned wisdom or lived experience, encourage them to challenge you. Make it safe by telling them that you welcome the opportunity for growth.

A wild idea

Many parents (but never you or me, of course) present their views as unquestionably correct. But children, no matter how young, are the experts on their own lives. They have earned wisdom about how to navigate their world. If we are to effectively guide them in the real world—*their* world—we must partner with them to gain an understanding of how we can best support them. What could be a better way of modeling intellectual humility than genuinely recognizing that our children can teach us? They are particularly well poised to guide us about how best to parent them. If you embrace this approach to parenting, I'll bet it will positively impact your relationship for decades.

Resources

Mark Leary. *The Psychology of Intellectual Humility*. John Templeton Foundation; 2018. https://www.templeton.org/wp-content/uploads/2020/08/JTF_Intellectual_Humility_final.pdf

This brief beautifully summarizes the science that demonstrates the importance of intellectual humility in building a citizenry better prepared to positively engage with each other.

Part 6

Preparation

I choose to be a Lighthouse Parent . . . I am committed to prepare them.

CHAPTER 28

From Toddlers to Teens: Supporting Their Need to Stand on Their Own

As a Lighthouse Parent, you strive to strike the balance between protecting your child (making sure they don't crash against the rocks) and preparing them to navigate the world on their own (riding life's waves). Your child is hardwired to learn to stand on their own even if their doing so activates your protective instincts. If you handle their inevitable march toward independence well, it will enhance your relationship with your child today, increase your influence during the teen years, and set the stage for a healthier connection throughout your lives.

Once independent, your child *can* stand on their own. It doesn't mean they *should* stand on their own. Being part of a community gives us a sense of belonging. Maintaining close relationships with extended family offers us comfort and security. The happiest people have interdependent lives with others they hold dear. Your adult child will most comfortably choose to remain connected to others if they can confidently navigate their own lives while simultaneously holding the desire to support others.

Your role now while raising a child is to support them as their independence blossoms and celebrate their ability to embark on new adventures. Let them know that as they grow, they have even more to contribute to our homes and in the world.

Preparing for Adolescence

Adolescents are wired to expand into new territories and strive to stand and run on their own. When you support this process, they invite guidance from you. When you resist their growing independence, they may reject your involvement in their life.

Shaping Your Lifelong Bond

Adult children welcome parents into their lives when they know their independence is respected. Their memories of you honoring their growing independence and decision-making during their childhood and adolescence will last forever.

But It's So Hard to Let Go...

We parents invest our heart and soul into a role that (many people think) disappears as our children grow. But our goal as Lighthouse Parents is different as we launch our children into their independent lives. Of course, we want our children to grow to think on their own and live satisfying and independent home and work lives. But we *also* hope that precisely because they can think and act independently, they confidently choose to benefit from sharing their lives with others, including us. I start with this point to address those butterflies in your belly signaling mixed feelings about your child's growing independence. You are not losing your child. You are gaining a thoughtful, confident adult child with whom you can maintain a strong relationship.

Nevertheless, many of us need to check in with ourselves to move past the discomfort that comes with our children asserting their independence. Let's consider 3 reasons why our children's road to independence leaves us ambivalent.

Raising a small child is joyful. This is true. We enjoy the time when our children are cute and consider us superheroes. It is hard to watch them grow up and to have our relationship become more complex. Try to look at it this way: as our children grow up there is more of them to love. And as they stop seeing us as superheroes it allows us to morph into real people. It is much easier to be a real person. Being a real human positions you to have the parent/adult-child relationship that allows you to rely on one another.

My job is to protect my child. Yes, it is. There is nothing more sacred than protecting a child when they are otherwise vulnerable. Ask any Mama lion or Papa bear. As your child grows you need to protect them in a different way. Overprotection backfires because it strongly communicates that you don't think your child can do it on their own. To fight your impulses of overprotection, repeat the following thoughts to yourself as often as needed:

- Preparation for the future is long-term protection.
- I want my child to make their mistakes under my watchful eye so I can help them recover and course correct.

"No" doesn't feel like a nice word. When your child was 2, they suddenly realized they had some choices. And they asserted themselves with this new sense of power. "No!" was a word you heard quite often. It seemed cute as their likes and dislikes began to surface. It is much less cute when our older children and adolescents assert themselves with their "noes!" Take a breath and remember that their ability to make choices and state their agreements and disagreements remains vital to learning to navigate the world on their own. And, while hearing "No!" doesn't feel nice to you, be glad for the fact your child can comfortably stand up for themselves. This will be protective when encountering negative influences in the world, as we will discuss in Chapter 30.

Preparation: one step at a time

Your child's development is full of firsts on the road to independence. Big momentous accomplishments. Their first steps. Their first words. Their first day at school. The first time they can go to the mall on their own. Their first date. The first time they turn the ignition key.

Some of these milestones will be met with or without your guidance. For example, you don't have to prepare your child to toddle those first steps. But most developmental milestones require some advanced skills and planning. These needn't feel as momentous if you've prepared your child with skills they need to conquer the task. Their first tween trip to the mall will go smoother if they already know not to be seduced by every sales gimmick, know the value of a dollar, and know how to contact you if they are in trouble. So think ahead of upcoming milestones and help your child build the necessary skills so they can more comfortably and successfully reach their goals.

Use your powers of observation as a first step to uncover the skills your child will need. You've got experience with this! When you childproofed your home, you imagined all the trouble your child could get into. You may even have gotten down on your knees to see the surroundings at toddler eye level. Now, give yourself a "child's-eye view."

Learning your child's perspective is easier than it was to imagine the world as a toddler. You don't have to get down on your knees. Your child has words! Remember they may not have a lot of experience, but they are the expert on their own life. Ask them to be a tour guide into their lives; this will bring your understanding of their needs to a new level. Once you understand the milestone they hope to achieve, ask them what they can handle now and what guidance or support they believe would be helpful. Then, join with them to develop a road map toward success. See this and other tips in the following table.

In *Letting Go With Love and Confidence: Raising Responsible, Resilient, Self-sufficient Teens in the 21st Century*, co-authored with Susan Fitzgerald, we address specific milestones and a stepwise approach to preparing our children for key milestones.

Say This (when supporting growing independence)	Not That
Show me what you can do.	You are not ready.
Tell me what you think.	I know _____.
You can handle a lot more than you used to be able to manage. What do you think you can do now?	You're too young.
Not yet. But I'll tell you what you've proven to me that you can handle.	No.
Yes. You've shown me you're ready for _____. Therefore, you can _____.	Yes.

Do This (when supporting growing independence)	Not That
Explain rules are in place because you care about safety.	Set rules with no explanation. Rules that are not understood feel like efforts to control rather than guide and protect.
Encourage your child to stretch into new territory.	Overprotect. This can instill a sense of fear of exploring the unknown.
Set clear boundaries around safety.	Trust blindly in your child's good judgment.

Say This (when supporting growing independence)	Not That
Recognize that your child having their own views is a critical step to them becoming their own person.	Disapprove of your child disagreeing with you.
Trust your child as the expert in their own life and seek advice from them about how much support you can give based on your earned wisdom and lived experience.	Communicate you've been through it all and understand how their life works better than they do.
Explain that boundaries can expand as children demonstrate they can handle more.	Make rigid boundaries. Children rebel against inflexible boundaries and may do so secretly.

Task accomplished, move on

Your child benefits when you prepare them for major steps in their life, but they must not see you as controlling their journey. They should see you as a guide who prepares them for their journey, not as somebody who smothers them with unneeded supervision. For example, your child needed you to teach them to tie their shoes. Once they learned, you didn't have to keep checking if their laces were tied. With that accomplished, it was time to move on to the next task.

Thinking for themselves

Watching your child develop into an independent thinker may be among the most thrilling aspects of parenting. Our child's thinking transforms from considering what they see into running with ideas that can change the world.

You can best support this amazing growth in your child's thinking by shifting from doing for your child to acting as a sounding board. Let them bounce off their thoughts and feelings. Create space for them to play out their plans. This helps them learn to make wise decisions, which is a critical skill that enables them to successfully stand on their own.

As your child develops into someone who can consider future possibilities, they can sometimes get ahead of themselves. Guide them to think more methodically by asking them questions about their plans. (Caution: Do this rarely, or it will feel like badgering. Most lessons they'll learn in the real world.) You'll use this strategy when your child comes to you for guidance or you sense they are struggling. Teach them how to make wise decisions and choose effective strategies by helping them to pause before putting their plans into action. Each stop along the way becomes an opportunity to consider possible consequences.

This approach aligns with what we discussed in Chapter 11 when we discussed "Working Toward That 'Aha!'"

If your child describes a plan that leaps from one idea to another, remain calm and help them settle their thoughts. Remember, frantic people can't think clearly. Then, invite them to consider the consequences of their initial thoughts versus what might happen if they approached their plan differently. This strategy of calmly pausing gives them the space to grasp that life does not precisely follow our plans. They'll learn to respond to changing realities and inevitable surprises. Stop at major decision points and ask them, "What do you think will happen now?" When they respond, help their thinking by saying, "What could you do if that did not happen to make it more likely things would go as you'd hope?" To help your child be ready to understand the importance of being responsive to changing circumstances, you might say, "But suppose that at this point, you hoped that _____ would happen but instead _____ happened?"

For example, shifting friendships can generate a rash response in middle school. Developing the skills to navigate human relationships well, and to avoid inflaming situations, is critical to managing the workplace as well as community and home relationships. Consider the following scenario:

Emily, a fifth grader, has a huge fight with her best friend, Jasmine, and now her entire group of friends is shunning her. Her first strategy, fueled by rage and the terror of rejection, is to share Jasmine's most intimidate secrets with the group. She thinks once the larger group knows these secrets, they will reject Jasmine and return to her. She tearfully shares this plan with her parent as she holds her phone in trembling hands, prepared to send out a group text. Her parent's protective instincts are on overdrive and therefore want to react angrily over Jasmine's betrayal.

But Emily's mother instead takes a breath, hugs and comforts her, gently removes the phone from her shaking hands, and says, "Let's think this through first and not send out a text while you're this upset."

Once Emily is no longer shaking, she asks her to consider what will happen if she presses send. Emily responds that the kids in her grade will all know "the truth" about Jasmine and that within minutes she'll have no friends. Then Jasmine will feel sorry that she turned the group against Emily. Her mother asks Emily what the group will think of her.

"What do you mean?" Emily asks.

"Well, do you think they will think you make a good, trusted friend?"

Emily experiences the aha that while embarrassing Jasmine, the group will also view Emily as a disloyal friend. With a little bit of time and prompting, she realizes that they will not choose her as a friend if she can't be trusted.

Her mother, asks, "Is there anything else you could do to help the group understand that they didn't treat you fairly, or even to make up with Jasmine?"

Emily responds, "Well, I don't even know why Jasmine got so mad at me. We've been friends since kindergarten, and we've had fights before but always made up."

Her mother gently prompts, "Could you write a different text asking Jasmine to talk with you about what started this? Maybe this will be just another fight between friends." This now becomes an opportunity for Emily to learn how to humbly communicate without escalating conflict.

Not all plans are emotionally driven; some are just hard to envision from the starting point. A young person might know their end goal and can state it clearly but has no idea that the journey is full of actions that can facilitate progress or generate roadblocks. Consequently, they have a goal but lack a strategy to achieve it. This can generate stress and does not help their road to independence. In these scenarios, it can help to break the journey into small manageable steps. Recall, that this is an essential strategy of managing stress. Point one: Identify and then address the problem (see Chapter 19).

Amir, a sixth grader, has big dreams. He has the intelligence to achieve them and remarkable drive for such a young man. But he is very disappointed in himself when he hits a roadblock and becomes derailed and often gives up. He then pretends he doesn't care and says things like, "That was a dumb idea anyway."

His parents know that Amir cares deeply and just needs better support in planning and needs to learn to be fueled by smaller achievements. Amir has long excelled in science and declares that he will win the science award this year by solving climate change. First, his parents reassure Amir that what makes them proud is his passion and the effort he puts into projects, not the award. They ask him what he will do to get started on his project. His initial response is that he'll just figure it out because he's frustrated the world's scientists haven't yet found the solution. Next, they talk about how science uncovers a small solution at a time and that real progress is made when added together with the work of others also trying to solve the problem. Knowing this, his parents ask him what his first step will be. Amir realizes that he can search the internet for ideas that people have already started on. Congratulating him for this initial step, his parents then ask what the next step would be. Amir says, "Well, when I find a scientist working on something I think is a great idea, maybe I can think about what I can do to help with that idea."

These strategies of helping your child be more thoughtful in their actions support your child to develop a growth mindset as detailed in Chapter 25. Recall that a growth mindset is key to your child being increasingly prepared to stand on their own because it helps them understand that their actions make a difference to their well-being, performance, and success. This approach of guidance helps your child slow their thinking and understand the consequences of their choices emphasizing that what they do creates their reality. Remember, you support a growth mindset when you help your child understand "I *did* _____ and therefore, _____ happened."

Parenting in this way helps your child absorb the lifelong lesson that receiving constructive feedback leads to a better outcome. This lesson will serve them well in college, the workplace, and in intimate relationships. Further, when children learn to exercise control in their lives, they see themselves as responsible for their own well-being and may be less likely to blame others for their struggles. This is core to resilience: when faced with challenges, children with a sense of control will be better prepared to take the action steps to bounce back.

Why Teens (*May Occasionally and Temporarily*) Reject Parents

Independence seeking takes on a sense of urgency to many adolescents. This can create painful parent-teen moments, full of noes and silences. It can feel like your child is pushing you away or even rejecting you. Trust me that they are not rejecting you; they are distancing themselves from the discomfort they feel about their reliance on you. Why are they uncomfortable? Their biological clock is telling them they will need to fly on their own, and they've grown comfortable living in the nest their parents have created for them. Their emotional and physical needs have been met. Deep down they wonder if they can do it on their own. To manage their discomfort, they must convince themselves they don't need you. Simply put, they push you away because they love you so much it hurts them.

How you handle this temporary phase will make a difference to your relationship. If you support your child to learn to stand on their own, they will grow to see you as a supportive guide in their journey. If you resent their efforts to become independent, find yourself hurt and angry, and restrict their attempts to stretch their wings, their resentment will deepen and could become long-lasting. My book *Congrats—You're Having a Teen! Strengthen Your Family and Raise a Good Person* helps you better understand your adolescent, including what drives their behavior. Its goal is to equip you with the knowledge and skill sets that will strengthen your relationship.

People Who Stand on Their Own Occasionally Fall

Our experience raising toddlers offers us lessons we can draw from throughout development as our children stumble. When toddlers fall on their bottoms the moment after they first stand up, they quickly glance toward their parents to know how they should respond. If their parents express alarm and run to help the little ones get back on their feet, toddlers cry and rely on their parents to pick them up. If, on the other hand, the parents say, "Bump! Get back up, little one," they learn that they have the power themselves to rise. Critically, they learn that although the power is theirs, encouragement helps.

CHAPTER 29

Communication: A Real-Life Skill

Our ability to communicate with one another with both our words and our steady, unwavering presence fosters the vital connections that enhance our sense of belonging. There may be nothing more protective, therefore, that you can do to prepare your child to thrive than to help them develop the communication skill sets that will ensure they maintain and develop healthy connections with others.

Given the centrality of human connection to our well-being and the importance of communication to maintaining those connections, this book is pretty much entirely about communication! This short chapter underscores key principles and reminds us that our childhood homes are where we learn how to interact with others. Therefore, how you communicate to your child is doing double duty; it guides and supports your child today *and* prepares them to interact with others throughout their lives.

Preparing for Adolescence

Adolescents may choose silence or distance as they work through their own thoughts and feelings. But if they have been raised with open communication that addresses thoughts and feelings, they'll know to share when they need you.

> ## Shaping Your Lifelong Bond
>
> Relationships that are forged with an understanding that listening is the cornerstone of support feel less pressure to get the words perfect. Rather they know that showing up—being present—is the key to communication. As your children become adults, you'll communicate your love to each other by showing up when needed.

We Hear, We Feel, We Pass It Along

As a Lighthouse Parent you strive to communicate your steadfast and reliable presence while also finding the right words to help shape your child into a person prepared to thrive. Because this book supports effective parenting, it guides you on what to say and do so your child feels heard, valued, protected, and prepared.

You're the model of an adult your child imagines becoming. Much of the way they communicate with others through their lifetimes will be rooted in how you communicate with them. Everything you do and say, through your words and attentive body language, teaches your child about human communication. Hopefully that means they will know how to be a reliable presence and support person for others.

The Essence of Effective Communication

Each of the chapters in the book offers specific communication strategies to position you as an effective Lighthouse Parent. In the following, I summarize some of the key elements of effective communication highlighted in this book. For each strategy, I could make the following statement: **Your child learns this (and any) communication skill best from watching you use it while experiencing its benefits.** For example, a child who is genuinely listened to feels heard. Feeling heard is such an affirming and empowering experience that once a person has felt the power and comfort of being heard, they'll always know that the starting point of effective communication is listening.

The following core elements of communication are not a complete list. Many have been touched on in previous chapters, while others are highlighted later in the book. Please consider other points you feel are critical to pass along to your child.

Be present. Words matter, but showing up speaks volumes. We communicate the unconditionality of our support by being there, especially in challenging times. When someone feels insecure, our unwavering presence lends them strength.

Get to calm first. During a challenging situation, humans go into fight, flight, or freeze mode. This diminishes the chances of successfully handling a challenge. We help people best when we first support them to settle their mind. We do this by lending them our calm—something we can only do when we take the steps first to calm ourselves.

Open communication. When we openly discuss thoughts and feelings it creates the opportunity to move forward, often with each other's support. On the other hand, when we don't discuss a topic, it tends to fester. In the case of mental health and emotional distress, choosing not to openly communicate sends the powerful message that the topic is one that holds shame or stigma.

Respectful listening. When we listen deeply while really hearing another person, they feel validated. That is the starting point to being able to offer supportive guidance or to communicate with someone about a subject that requires collaboration or compromise.

Listening with humility. We'll never grow if we don't consider new ideas. We'll also never gain from others' wisdom or experience if we are not hearing their views with an open and curious mindset. In the case of raising children, this takes on urgency. We can only guide them if we learn from them what their lives look like. Seeing our children as experts in their own life is not a slogan; it is a strategic first step to understanding how best to support them.

Speaking when asked. People communicate when they are ready for guidance. If you jump in too quickly with advice before a person is ready to hear it, they may not be receptive to your wisdom.

Keep it strength-based when promoting progress. Nobody wants to be fixed or to be viewed through a lens of brokenness. The secret to guiding someone to live to their potential is to use their existing strengths as a foundation to launch a discussion.

Influencing wisely. Nobody likes it when other people interfere in their personal business or try to micromanage their lives. But people genuinely value others caring about their well-being. When we frame our guidance to be about safety or our concern for their well-being or success, our thoughts are welcomed.

Respectful guidance. When we recognize a person's expertise in what navigating their life looks and feels like and have gotten permission to offer guidance, we will proceed respectfully in sharing our thoughts and recommendations.

Being a self-advocate. People must learn to stand up for themselves without putting another person down. The first step is to understand when someone else is trying to assert positive or negative influence. The next step is to thoughtfully and respectfully assert what you know is best for your own well-being.

The language of humility and forgiveness. There is an art to restoring relationships that have been damaged. It is about listening respectfully, humbly asking for forgiveness when necessary, and reinforcing the importance of the relationship.

Communication Strategies That Must Be Preserved in a Changing World

Although most communication skills are best shown when modeled, there are some points that need to be explicitly stated in a changing communication landscape.

Thoughts communicated through social media live forever. Blowing off steam has an entirely new meaning now. Words that may have been easily forgotten in the past live forever on the internet. We all must take a deep breath and pause before sharing our feelings with the world, including any future employers.

There are real people on the other end of our virtual communications. People have gotten so used to freely sharing their opinions instantly through emojis, likes, and dislikes that they seem to forget that actual humans receive these notes of affirmation or disdain. Furthermore, the algorithms seem to be designed to respond to our opinions with information that only reinforces them. This divides us and only reinforces and hardens our stances. It has made some people feel they are entitled to belittle those who disagree and feel safe doing so behind a screen. The bottom line is real people with real feelings can get hurt by online communications.

Texting and virtual communication do not replace person-to-person communication. Many young people consider face-to-face communication awkward and inefficient. They have seen that texting allows them to make their point and even express their emotions fluidly and with little thought. We must ensure that our children never lose those critical in-person communication skills, such as a warm handshake, looking respectfully at someone, and stating their thoughts clearly. Keeping people away from virtual communication is not an option. However, we can ensure "protected time" for real communication with phones away. We must continue to teach human-to-human skill sets. You want your child to grow to be someone who can look a potential employer in the eye and say, "I'm the right person for this position and I'll commit to learning and growing on the job." You want them to be someone who can wrap their arms around a distressed friend and say "I'm not going anywhere."

A Lighthouse Communicates...

The lighthouse metaphor may be best understood by what a real lighthouse communicates. It's there for safety and guidance. It is a beacon that helps you navigate the waters more confidently because you can always look back to collect your bearings. It is a trusted, reliable presence.

CHAPTER 30

Influence You Can Trust: Assessing Misinformation and External Pressure

Forces that influence our thoughts and actions can come from many directions. As parents, we must prepare our children by guiding them to think for themselves, assess potential influences for accuracy, and consider the intent of those delivering information to them. This is one more case, however, where your loving presence is both the best protection for your child today and what positions you to prepare them for the future. Your knowledge of your child's core values reinforces their strength to stand by their convictions, defend themselves against harmful influences, and resist undermining messages.

Preparing for Adolescence

You want your child to think for themselves, while also having your protective voice playing in their heads. You can guide them how to assess other forces trying to influence them while knowing that (even though you won't always get it right) you'll always have their best interest in mind.

Shaping Your Lifelong Bond

Lifelong trust forms when your child knows that no matter how complex the world may be or how many forces try to gain influence over them, they can always count on you considering only what is best for them.

Peer Influence—For Better or Worse

Forming close peer relationships is an important part of human development. These relationships teach children how to work together as well as how to stand up for themselves. These are critical skills in the workplace and are the roots of collaboration and self-advocacy. It is with peers that children also form the kind of trusting, intimate relationships that are the foundation of healthy romantic partnerships.

Knowing how critical peer relationships are to human development, it comes as no surprise that they are deeply influential. Because children want to fit in with their peers, they are likely to want to do the same thing that "everyone" is doing. Breathe. This is not necessarily a bad thing. Peers taking school seriously, contributing to the community, helping their families function, displaying teamwork on the court or field, or creativity in the arts, are a positive influence on your child. On the other hand, peers engaging in worrisome behaviors also can influence your child. This makes your role clear—have your child hang out with positive influencing peers. If only it were that simple. You *can* be a positive influence that makes it more likely your child will have positive peers and be prepared to recognize and respond to negative influences.

How we handle peer influence in childhood will pay off most noticeably in the teen years when adolescents search for their new group in preparation for eventually leaving our homes. Help your child learn to manage peer relationships in childhood, while they are listening to you on this matter, so that peer management will be in their existing repertoire. If you focus on it too much in adolescence you will be entering their "personal" territory and your advice may backfire. However, you will always be welcome to talk about peers, or anything else, if you make it clear you are doing so because of a safety concern.

Supporting positive peer relationships

Friends who make wise choices for themselves will encourage your child to do the same. Positive peers can also gently push your child to build confidence to stretch themselves. They may also encourage your child to give up bad habits and consider healthier ones. Authentic friends support each other to get through hardships and celebrate their strengths together. For all these reasons, you hope your child will benefit from being surrounded by positive, meaningful friendships. While you can't, and shouldn't, choose their friends, you can increase the chances they will have positive connections. Consider the following strategies:

Encourage varied activities. Children who participate in structured programs have improved academic performance and better physical health and are less likely to engage in risky behaviors. These are good places to build positive friendships.

Encourage multiple peer groups. Children should have more than one group of friends. They can be drawn from the family, school, neighborhood, clubs, sports, or religious settings. This ensures that when relationships become rocky in one group your child will not suffer from isolation because they can turn to another circle of friends. Further, if a group turns toward undesired behaviors, your child will feel less pressure to follow their path if they have friendship choices.

Be welcoming and present without hovering. Knowing who your child is spending time with offers you a window into their life without being intrusive. Keep your house stocked with healthy snacks, and let your child make your house a comfortable and welcoming place for friends. Then, observe the friendship dynamics.

Make it easy to do the right thing

Agree on common rules with your child's friends' parents. If a group of friends have parents with shared protective boundaries, they'll more comfortably follow the expected rules.

Minimizing undesired peer influences
Let's become grounded in the big picture.

- Your child (and future tween, teen, and adult) will be more likely to follow their own values when they know what matters to them. Help them clarify what they care about and who they want to be. Supporting their development of a sense of meaning and purpose will help them stick to their goals.
- Ensuring they feel secure in your unwavering love will position you (forever!) as a person whom they can always turn to for a gut check. Your child will make mistakes because they are human. They'll want to course correct but may need guidance how to shift directions. If they know you may disapprove of a behavior but never reject them, they'll turn to you for guidance.

- If your child knows you'll be a sounding board about personal matters and comment only when asked but steer them quickly from danger, they'll check in with you.
- If your child knows that even if they come to you troubled by a friend's behavior, you'll judge the action and not the friend (unless true danger presents), you'll more likely know their social landscape and be positioned to offer guidance.

All of this is best accomplished in calm moments when you can help your child build their decision-making muscles, rather than in a heated moment when a BIG decision is imminent. Our goal is for them to have a clear sense of what matters to them and to know they should always turn to those values when making decisions rather than make choices when under pressure.

Peer navigation skills
We can help our children build 4 skill sets to manage peer influence.

- Recognizing manipulation.
- Successfully navigating around undermining influence.
- Learning to say "no!" effectively.
- Shifting the blame to adult supervision.

Recognizing Manipulation

Peer influence is usually subtle and often does not even involve words. In fact, it can be internally driven: "I'll fit in if I just show them that I'm like them," or, "They'll like me more if I prove I'm brave." Insecurity rises regardless of our values when we seek acceptance.

But sometimes it is others who intentionally subtly or blatantly manipulate our children. Your child must first recognize they are being manipulated and then draw from a practiced vocabulary to respond. These words must be practiced because when people are stressed they can't think creatively or wisely. You might get away with role-playing with your child but will unlikely engage your tween or teen in "awkward" role-plays. Instead, leverage teachable moments. For example, when driving past a group of youth vaping, you might say, "That boy looks about 11 and is engaging in a dangerous habit. How do you think he started vaping?" A child or pre-tween may assume he was forced or tricked into it. This enables you to say that while some kids might feel forced, many might do it just to fit in. In this low-pressure setting, you can help your child consider better ways to fit in and strategies to avoid situations where they might experience pressure. And you can help them develop scripts to respond to pressure.

Successfully Navigating Around Undermining Influence

Because peers are so important to our children, we must teach them how to control their own actions while maintaining friendships. This strategy has 3 stages.

- **Stage 1:** Your child needs to recognize when they are being manipulated. You can teach them how people subtly influence others even while staying away from personal situations. You might consider scrolling the internet and discussing pop-up advertisements, walking through a store and discussing sales techniques, or witnessing child or teen behaviors when in a group.
- **Stage 2:** Your child can be guided to state their positions firmly and clearly without being angry, hostile, or belittling. "I'm not going to tease that new kid." "I'm not cheating."
- **Stage 3:** They can then offer an alternative plan that allows them to maintain the relationship on their terms. "I think he's new here and doesn't know the kind of things we like. Let's invite him to sit with us and see where he's from." "I'm pretty good at math; I'll help you figure out how to solve these problems."

Learning to Say "No!" Effectively

When the word "no" is used casually or too often, it loses its power. When said while smiling, "no" is interpreted as "Ask me again, it'll become a yes." Many children don't like to say "no" because "it sounds mean." Guide your child that clear responses avoid confusion and allow them to choose what they do.

Shifting the Blame to Adult Supervision

Even when children know what they should do, it is difficult to take a stand if it differs from what their peers are doing. You can help your child get out of challenging situations while still fitting in. The following 2 strategies offer a way your child can choose to do the right thing by shifting blame to you. These strategies summon the supervision you want to give to them.

The check-in rule

The check-in rule is a bedtime routine to be used every night, no exceptions. In childhood you create the habit that your child must say goodnight to you. Even if your tween or teen rolls their eyes, never loosen this expectation. Bedtime is a great time to create space for discussions. Your child always knows that if they need you, you'll be there. It also helps children "call in your watchful eyes" as needed. *"Are you kidding? I'd never get away with that. We have to talk every night, so they'd find out!"*

Code words

Choose a code word or phrase your child can use to signal for your supervision when they need to leave a risky or uncomfortable social situation. They call or text you presumably to ask permission, but casually insert the code. *"Yeah, I won't be home so I can't help you change the sparkplugs tonight."* (Sparkplugs is the code.) Alerted to a difficult situation, you demand your child comes home. If they can get home safely, they leave while complaining about how strict you are. If they can't get home on their own, they could say, *"Well, I would but my ride can't leave yet."* Then, arrange a pick-up. Two points: 1) Change the code word; you can only change sparkplugs so often ☺. 2) If you want your child to use this potentially life-saving strategy, state in advance that you'll be grateful and relieved if they reach out to you for help, and they'll never be punished for the trouble they found themselves in.

Social Media and Virtual Pressure

Fitting in has taken on a whole new meaning in the digital age. The virtual world provides young people opportunities to create and recreate different versions of themselves. All of this is potentially wonderful because nobody has to feel alone. That can be deeply protective for people who don't easily fit in. In today's virtual world, there is a mutual support group for every young person.

But the virtual world also creates a new source of undermining influence. Before we let our children navigate these barely charted waters alone, we need to prepare our children to protect themselves. To do so, we need to keep abreast of the rapidly changing landscape of virtual communication. The following highlights essential discussions to have with your child about the virtual world:

The virtual world is a false reality. Many people are inauthentic online. They glamorize their life, alter their appearances, and pretend to be eternally joyful. This can hurt our children in 2 ways. First, if they post an inauthentic portrayal of themselves, they may subconsciously create an internal dialogue that suggests the true version of themselves would be unacceptable. Second, they might fail to notice that the online lives they scroll through are not real. This makes them vulnerable to being influenced by the false belief that they would be happier if only they looked or acted a certain way.

Avoid having FOMO change your habits. The virtual world never sleeps. This makes young people live with FOMO or fear of missing out. The pace of information bombarding them influences them to forgo rest and attempt to keep up.

Online popularity is not the real thing. Virtual popularity is measured by emojis, likes, retweets, and views. In fact, many online influencers earn their popularity through absurd behaviors and outrageous views. In the real world, people foster connections through mutual support. We need to reinforce that we must behave in the real world in a way that builds our communities, fosters real relationships, and strengthens our families.

Dangerous people are often the best at engaging others online. Young people can fall prey to others taking advantage of their vulnerability. People can find support groups that reinforce undermining beliefs about themselves or radicalize them by welcoming them into countercultural groups. Tragically, we must also prepare our children to be vigilant and skeptical of the type of flattery predators use to influence and engage vulnerable youth. This is a "putting your hand on the stove moment" where you cannot allow any room for error. Children must learn they should never respond online to a person who asks them to send pictures or meet them in person. Reinforce the idea that they should always come to you with any suspicious people or activity and that they'll never get in trouble when they come to you to stay safe.

Misinformation and orchestrated divisiveness

Media literacy has taken on a sense of urgency in these divisive times. It used to be clear where trusted information could be found. Now some people (or bots!) intentionally spread disinformation through the digital space. Lies can feel very much like truths when repeated often enough or spoken with conviction. Dangerous content can contain enough engaging points and accurate information to draw people in and then change direction and expose them to sexist, racist, anti-LGBTQIA+, anti-Semitic, or Islamophobic tropes. This story is old; what is terrifyingly new is how easily hatred spreads and how rapidly it can disrupt our society.

We must have hard conversations with our children about navigating these issues. And we must keep abreast of a rapidly changing landscape so we can keep our conversations current and share how we seek credible information. The following concepts are discussions we start gently in childhood while our children are still closely supervised and that intensify with our adolescents as they navigate digital spaces more independently.

People spread false information, sometimes intentionally, sometimes through error. There is a difference between misinformation and disinformation. The American Psychological Association clarifies that "misinformation is a mistake," but "disinformation is deliberate." Many people or groups want to shape or influence opinions and may mistakenly spread false information. Sometimes, however, content is meant to turn people against one another. Sadly, it can make people less likely to resolve conflicts and to instead move into their respective corners.

Just because you see it all over social media doesn't mean it's true. Today's algorithms create infinite realities. Once we click on something that looks intriguing it changes how the algorithm understands us. We receive more related information; then, too often, a radical notion will be inserted into the content, potentially drawing us into a cycle of radicalization and further division.

What enrages, engages. Your child will likely ask, "Why would people do this? Don't they know they are lying?" I defer to your deep knowledge of your child on how to explain that some hurting people are driven by hatred. We can tell them that although we may never understand people's motivations, we must choose to build strong communities and respect and care for each other. We can also explain that sometimes people think the best way to get you on their side is to make you move away from hearing other viewpoints. The simplest thing to explain is people make money off our rage. As we become enraged, we click more, and they earn more.

The following list of media literacy questions were proposed by Eden Pontz, the executive producer and director of digital content for the Center for Parent and Teen Communication (https://parentandteen.com) to help families discern credible information from misinformation or disinformation. I suggest you work through these questions with your own child.

- Does this content encourage an extreme reaction from you? (For example, if it makes you angry or scared, that should be a red flag.)
- Who is the author or creator?
- Who is the target audience?
- What is the source of the information and what do you know about this source? (Are they a credible journalist or organization or artificial intelligence? Do they have biases or an agenda that is shaping the imformation?)
- What is the motivation behind sharing this information?
- What qualifications do the experts included in the content have?
- Does the content provide evidence for what's being said? (Does that evidence make sense?)
- Is the website URL legitimate? Or is it subtly changed to make you believe you are going to a credible source while directing you instead to disinformation?
- If content takes you to a website, how does it look? (For example, are there grammatical errors, words in all caps, claims with no sources, or sensationalized images?)
- Is there anything missing from the message? (And if so, might it be important to include?)
- What makes you think this is credible?
- Is this content a joke? (Did it come from a humorous website, for example?)

Using the virtual world as an information source can be deeply confusing. Model using sites that check credibility and offer lessons on media literacy. In the most heated time consider turning off the devices!

Parenting Matters

Your influence over your child is not in competition with peer or media influence. Your unconditional love remains the critical influence that shapes how they see themselves. And your guidance remains the most effective way for them to learn to navigate other influences in their lives. I promise.

Resources

Digital Wellness Lab. This site offers parents the latest science-based resources to learn what you need to know about a specific type of technology or how media can affect children's and adolescents' health and well-being. https://digitalwellnesslab.org

Common Sense Media. Media and technology are at the center of kids' lives every day. With more and more of life happening online, what catches kids' attention isn't always what's best for them, and what companies do with their personal information isn't always clear. Since 2003, Common Sense Media has been the leading source of entertainment and technology recommendations for families and schools. https://www.commonsensemedia.org

Part 7
Reliability

I choose to be a Lighthouse Parent . . . I'll remain a source of light they can seek whenever they need a safe and secure return.

CHAPTER 31

Creating a Family Culture
of Forgiveness

None of our homes are stress free. Sometimes the world's negative stress seeps through our walls and puts us on edge, affecting our behavior with one another. Sometimes it is precisely because of how much we care for our loved ones that we find ourselves upset about something we'd barely notice in someone else. Or we care so deeply that we become particularly frustrated when one of us makes a mistake. The point is our homes are complicated places where we are not always on our best behavior. As a result, we can hurt or disappoint each other.

You have committed to creating a home that remains a stable source of security. That becomes more critical during stressful times. Our homes must remain a source of light our children can seek whenever they need a safe and secure return. This means that our love remains unconditional, and no words spoken or actions taken, by anybody, will create a permanent schism in our relationships. We must create a culture of forgiveness in our homes that is so entrenched that none of us need ever fear rejection. Such a culture ensures we'll be there for each other when we are most needed.

Preparing for Adolescence

You never know when your adolescent will need you most. But you want to be sure they come to you when they do. If they fear rejection, they may choose not to share what is troubling them. If your family has a culture of forgiveness, you are more likely to know what is going on in your child's life because they needn't fear losing you.

Shaping Your Lifelong Bond

We, parents and adult children, will all make mistakes throughout our lives. Nothing should fracture our relationships. Families with a culture of forgiveness can move past inevitable rough patches. Especially when we feel judged by others, families should remain a safe harbor.

An Imperfect Person in an Imperfect Family

It starts with humility. The only way we can be forgiving of one another (and of ourselves) is if we draw comfort from our humanity. None of us will ever get it all right. We are works in progress. Many of us let our game faces down in our homes because we feel safest there; we do not need to pretend that we are handling life with ease. And most of us experience our greatest frustrations in situations we care most about—meaning our family members can potentially cause us the greatest grief. Only once we acknowledge the imperfection that comes with being human can we create a culture of forgiveness. Your child will be spared a lot of despair over their lifetime if they assess their own imperfections in the context of knowing we all need second chances. Critically, knowing they have a second chance, they'll seek opportunities to right their wrongs rather than deny their problems.

Why a Culture of Forgiveness Protects Your Child

Creating a home with a culture of forgiveness offers protection for your child now and throughout their lives. Furthermore, it protects your relationship far into the future. Let's briefly consider why. Some of the following thoughts underscore points made throughout this book:

- Success rises from failure. With each failure we take a second (and third, and fourth . . .) chance to get it better. If people fear failure, they forgo this opportunity for growth.
- Your child will come to you only when they know that doing so will bring support and guidance rather than risk rejection. As discussed in Chapter 5, judgments of any kind instill a fear in your child that they, too, might be rejected. A culture of forgiveness does the opposite.
- Many young people make behavioral mistakes, even risky ones, as they grow. They'll need guidance to course correct. They won't seek that guidance if they know they'll get in trouble for their disclosure. If, on the other hand, they know they'll be forgiven and guided toward safety, they'll see disclosure as a first step forward. This is how we are positioned to support positive behavioral changes and safe choices.
- The world may often be unforgiving and sometimes doesn't give second chances. Our children must know throughout their lives that there are ALWAYS opportunities to make amends and to grow from a mistake. At the very least, they must know that they will never be rejected by family. That ensures you and your child an irreplaceable relationship throughout life.
- Our children must know we will never give up on them. Once they think that we have lost hope in them, they might give up on themselves, feeling they have nothing to lose. "After all," they might think, "my family doesn't think I'm much good anyway, so I may as well do what they expect from me." This can be the start of a downward spiral. We prevent this undermining thinking by holding our children to being their best selves and always expecting them to return to their core values. This is also how we help our children return to us even after they've endured difficult times, as we discuss in Chapter 33.

What does a home with a culture of forgiveness look like?

A home steeped in the culture of forgiveness approaches life with humility knowing that we are all on a journey with lessons to be learned and mistakes to be gotten past. To be clear, it is not a perfect place; it is a place where growth is allowed. It is a place where relationships are held as sacred and that people do the intentional work of resolving tension. No deed or word spoken in frustration or anger holds more power than the core of the relationship.

People still get hurt in homes with a culture of forgiveness. People still make mistakes there. But when they do, they don't hear something like, "This is what I've grown to expect." Instead, they learn that their family remains committed to knowing we all can do better and are more likely to get there with each other's support.

Am I allowed to be critical?

Yes. Being nonjudgmental does not mean you don't care or notice a problem. In fact, your sulking or stewing in silence just intensifies a child's fear of disappointing you and increases their anxiety that trouble is brewing. Being forgiving does not mean you aren't hurt. It means you focus on the problem the other person can solve, rather the person themselves being the problem. It means you see the problem as a mistake that they can solve based on their existing strengths. When you are critical, you can be so while emphasizing you care and expressing the confidence that this mistake can be overcome.

Parents practice self-compassion

I'll bet that you're expecting me to use this opportunity to again extol the benefits of self-compassion for parents and caregivers. Good (educated) guess! If you're consistently hard on yourself despite being generous with your forgiveness toward others, your forgiving gestures toward your child won't be believed. In fact, if you experience your child's mistakes as yet another sign that you are an ineffective parent, your child may experience anxiety because they see their actions as hurting your belief in yourself.

Care for yourself as you care for others. Forgive your own mistakes. Know that others' mistakes are rarely a reflection of you. This is healthy for you and makes you the kind of parent who will be invited to guide your child as they grow through their challenges.

Modeling and talking

Like all aspects of parenting, we teach best when we model the behavior we hope to see in our children. In this case, when our children see us practicing self-forgiveness and witness us forgiving our life partners, friends, relatives, and colleagues, they see how much smoother relationships become. Further, they see our emotional burden lessened as we let go of some our own anger. Most significantly, as they benefit from your forgiveness, they experience enhanced security and want to pass that along to others.

However, learning to genuinely earn forgiveness requires some coaching. Let's explore that word "earn." A young child thinks one word alone suffices to earn forgiveness, but our adolescents need to have a far more sophisticated understanding. We coach our children at a developmentally appropriate level responding to their growing capability of gaining a deeper understanding of what merits genuine forgiveness.

Our young children quickly learn the power of the word "sorry." We first let them know when they did something wrong. We then told them that they needed to say, "I'm sorry." When they followed our instructions, we reinforced their action by hugging them and saying, "I forgive you." We coached them to understand this.

The next step is for our children to understand how their actions impact others. We coach them to understand this when we say something like, "Do you see that you hurt Lydia's feelings? Please say that you're sorry to Lydia." This is a critical step to them gaining empathy and to understanding that their words and actions can both hurt and be used to heal. We help them understand their actions affect us when we avoid using an accusatory tone such as, "You made me feel _____!" Instead, we need to draw their empathy, "I feel like _____ when _____ happens." This naturally generates reflection and will likely trigger the response, "I didn't mean to _____. I'm sorry."

We want our older children to grow to understand that the word "sorry" should signal a plan for change and growth. They must first demonstrate that they understand they have done something to warrant offering an apology. Then, they must learn that genuine forgiveness is earned when we both own our mistake and arrive at a plan to do better. We can coach them to grasp this when we state, "You made a mistake. There is no reason to dwell on this. I want you to think through the lesson you've learned. More importantly, let's think through what action you can take to do better next time. I love you. Thanks for telling me about this and choosing to include me in your life."

A believable apology

We can model and teach our children that a genuine apology makes it clear that a lesson has been learned. It takes responsibility for any harm that may have been caused, whether intentional or not. It explains what will be done to make up for the mistake and that you hope to avoid repeating the mistake. This is best done when we tie together the apology, an understanding of the deed, and the solution. "I'm sorry I came home late. I understand why you were worried. I will call next time."

Genuine forgiveness

It may be that offering forgiveness is harder than offering an apology. Neither generating guilt nor expressing disappointment is productive. You may state what went wrong. But focus on what can improve the situation. Forgiveness does not imply you have forgotten the behavior. (In fact, you should stay alert for the behavior's recurrence.) Rather, it states that you are willing to move on and find a better path forward.

When your child experiences the profound relief that comes from feeling forgiven, they will want to continue to please you. Most critically, they will continue to include you in their life even when they are feeling embarrassed or ashamed because they know your relationship is unshakable.

CHAPTER 32

Weathering Relationship Challenges and Rebuilding Trust

A Lighthouse Parent demonstrates their reliability best during a storm. When you realize your family is not functioning as it should, it doesn't mean you've failed. In sharp contrast, you are courageous and committed if you recognize that the relationships in your home need a reset to change dysfunctional patterns. You know your family is worth investing in and that change is possible. Moreso, when you demonstrate that the price of maintaining healthy families is hard work, you prepare your child to have more successful relationships throughout their life. Perhaps above all, when your child sees that your family members work hard to maintain and restore relationships, they learn that tough times may hit, but recovery is possible. And that while we don't look for challenges, when we work through them, we can draw closer.

Preparing for Adolescence

Most adolescents will not engage in risky behaviors, but some will. Many adolescents will push their parents away temporarily as they try on different hats and stretch toward an independence that both excites and intimidates them. You will get through these times if you are equipped with an understanding that family bonds should never be broken and that there are always opportunities to rebuild a warm and trusting relationship.

Shaping Your Lifelong Bond

When relationships outside our families are challenged, human bonds may become broken beyond repair. Families are special. Our bonds should offer unshakable security; they should be seen as unbreakable. As clear as this sounds, it is not easy, and we all know families that no longer function. We must be intentional about maintaining our relationships. As we raise our children, we can set the stage for a communication style that ensures our relationships will weather future strains.

Families Deserve a Growth Mindset

In Chapter 25, we discussed how a growth mindset promotes thriving in an individual, largely because they see themselves as capable of changing and welcome feedback from others on how to improve. Recall that when we speak in a way that suggests our children *are* something we set our expectations (and theirs) that they will remain that way. You *are* lazy. You *are* selfish. Or even, you *are not* good at math. Instead, when we comment on their actions, what they *do*, we remind them they can grow if they put in the effort.

Our families deserve a growth mindset. They can change. When we stop labeling them in their entirety as dysfunctional and instead highlight specific things not going as well as we'd hope, we promote a family growth mindset. We are not broken. We are engaging in a behavior, one we can change when we put in the intentional effort to break a cycle. We can endure rough times if we have the mindset to continue to grow; the language to reengage in caring, open communication; and the commitment to rebuilding trust.

Relationships Are Sacred

Remember that tension can boil over in our homes precisely because they are safe spaces to let it all out. And we are most likely to be angry or disappointed by the actions of people we care most about. This can feel like it threatens our relationships, but resolving these tensions proves our relationships are secure. Yes, families are complicated, but it is in our families that we learn that you can have conflict and recover. We can be temporarily (or maybe longer) unpleasant and still be cared about. When our families are stretched to their limits but we continue to support each other, we demonstrate the sacred nature of unwavering love.

Dialing down the temperature

When people speak of "dialing down the temperature" during stressful inter-actions, they usually mean taking a breath, removing yourself from a situation, and choosing to address it when calmer. These strategies prevent us from reacting out of anger. I am more interested, however, in taking the temperature way down to catalyze the reset necessary to invest in the hard work of repairing the relationship. Certainly, there are crises that deserve immediate attention and may not allow time for that breath, but most relationship challenges are better approached when grounded in the inherent strength of your relationship.

Remember high-yield time

When there is a relationship challenge, the air feels thick and people presume that every time you're together the focus will be on challenging topics. This increases tension and does little to underscore the security from which problems are best addressed. Spend some time just enjoying each other. There will be time and a space for discussion. This is the highest-yield strategy to ultimately resolve conflict. In fact, make it explicit. Say, "Let's go out and enjoy time together. I promise not to have any heavy discussions. I just want to be with you."

Falling back in (unconditional) love

Every time you hear me speak (endlessly) about the critical nature of unconditional love, remind yourself that you are allowed to not like something someone you love does. It's hard to be unconditionally loving when you're frantic or angry. Your goal is to ensure your relationship is maintained and ultimately strengthened because together you have endured these challenges. Knowing how badly your love is needed by your loved one doesn't make it easy to move past your justified emotions, but it does help you know in your gut that there is no other path.

Remind yourself why you feel so strongly. It is the depth of your love that makes you so full of feelings. Allow yourself to focus on your loved one's strengths, as we discuss more fully in the next chapter. Reflect on all the reasons that the person angering you today has earned your love. Bathe in those feelings. Launching from this loving space, one that cannot change, you can more calmly approach what it is that you are not liking.

Getting on the same page

Let's assume in this part that a child or adolescent's undesirable behavior is the primary family stressor. It is critical that all the caring adults be on the same page. You must be intentional about coming together as a family unit because turmoil could too easily push you apart. If your response is not unified, one adult may become labeled as "nice" while the other is seen as too strict, overly controlling, or insensitive. This can be the starting point for our children to learn to further drive the divisions because it may ease the consequences they receive. These manipulative behaviors driven by the child, coupled with the disagreements over parenting, can split families apart.

First, wrestle through ideas together as adults before you approach your child. It is better to present a unified compromise than to parent with opposing viewpoints. This will leave less space for manipulation and will spare your child the anxiety that comes with needing to process mixed messages. Good, unified messages include

- You care about this because you love your child.
- You are committed to keeping them safe.
- You care that they possess the kind of character strengths that ensure success in the future.
- You disapprove of the current undesired behavior because it interferes with one of the previous points or has consequences for family function.

- You have agreed on a consequence that is designed to teach them the importance of not repeating the mistake.
- You continue to see them as a good person and this mistake does not change that in any way.
- There is a path to completely re-earning your trust.

Places and Spaces

When you're approaching a hard topic, do so in a way that respects privacy and prevents public embarrassment. Remembering what you felt like as a child, and especially a teen, will help you have important conversations and even offer corrections without overwhelming or shaming your child. The following tips also likely apply to tough adult-to-adult conversations:

1. Start conversations low key. If you begin too emotionally, it makes children uncomfortable, and many teens squirm. Sometimes it makes them worry about you, making them feel they need to take care of you. That makes it harder for them to problem-solve.
2. Never have hard conversations in public.
3. Never have hard conversations in front of friends.
4. Don't start difficult conversations when someone is already emotionally overloaded about another topic. If they are upset about the topic at hand, it's appropriate to proceed after lowering the temperature.
5. On the other hand, if they are finally relaxed after a difficult day or stressful period, consider postponing the conversation long enough for them to catch their breath.

Communication pearls for tough topics

Reinforce family culture of forgiveness
A heartfelt and meaningful apology offers a reset. Sometimes it is enough. Other times harm has been done, and an apology is only a starting point. Even then, a commitment of forgiveness is the underpinning of progress in a strained relationship (as discussed in Chapter 31).

An us problem, not a you problem

Nobody wants to feel as though they are the source of problems. In most cases, particularly those that involve interactions, we all could do better. Further, any solutions must include everyone involved. If a solution suggests only one person makes changes, they will feel labeled as the problem and that will curtail progress.

Prevent unspoken signals from conflicting with your words

Remain rooted in your caring. Truly believe in progress. Otherwise, your body and facial expressions will display your true feelings—disdain or hopelessness—and will undermine your words. Our bodies convey the truth and speak volumes. It's hard work to remain eternally hopeful. When possible, do the reflective work that helps you get past your pessimism or catastrophic thinking before you directly address concerns with another person.

Sometimes being friendly is not what's needed

We all want to be liked. Sometimes during stressful times with our children or other adults, we double down on our friendliness. Friends are critical people in our lives, but they are not always reliable. Family must be. So, when we overplay the friend card, we unintentionally diminish the depth of our reliability. Be family. Solid. Unwavering in your presence.

Highlight importance not urgency

As urgent as a matter may feel, approach it as though it is important, but not as though you are in a crisis. Otherwise, you'll activate the stress hormones that prevent the rational thought and emotional intelligence you all need to move forward. Remind yourself no solution rides on any one conversation. This will allow you to stay calmer and focus on everyone feeling heard and supported.

Don't start by undermining growth

When we are most frustrated with one another, words sometime blurt out of our mouths that halt any potential for conversation. "You always ___." "You never ___." "This is exactly what I've learned to expect from you." "You have no idea. No idea." These kinds of phrases suggest no potential for change. Pinch yourself if you must, but don't use these phrases. If they slip out because they are scripts replaying from your own childhood, apologize and start over.

Don't make assumptions

Sometimes we assume too much about what another person is thinking. Or think we fully understand the words they are saying. We also tend to trust that we are correctly interpreting unspoken cues. However, we are often mistaken and therefore waste the potential to problem-solve. Avoid this trap by checking on your assumptions. Share your understanding and welcome a correction. You might say, "If I am hearing you correctly, it seems you might be feeling _____; am I right?" In parallel, try not to predict how others are experiencing your thoughts or feelings. Help them out. Be clear about your thoughts and your needs and tell people what kind of response would be most meaningful to you.

Not everything needs to be said

Sharing every concern, terror-filled fantasy, and lingering grudge is not necessary. In fact, it might backfire because it creates that sense of urgency as previously described and leads to others not hearing you. Further, if you focus on your hurt, it can make it feel as though you care most about your pain, rather than repairing your relationship or steering your child (or other adult) toward wiser behaviors. And, if you focus only on your pain, you'll make others withhold information from you to spare you more pain. Thus, say what you need to say to initiate progress. But some feelings can be left unsaid.

Facilitate, don't dictate

When we talk at someone it drives them away. We engage them when we talk with them. So, share your thoughts and feelings, but never forget that your intention is to engage the other person to access their thoughtfulness and decision-making skills. So, listen. Then guide them one step at a time.

Listening and talking

People don't share all their thoughts or allow their feelings to unfold if the person they are talking to reacts before they feel heard. How you listen creates safety for another person to share their vulnerability. And, in turn, how you talk determines whether you will be listened to. Giving directives causes people to tune out and can breed resentment. Engaging with them in a back-and-forth while being flexible to hearing their view encourages them to hear you and be less entrenched in their thinking.

I, not you

An "I" statement gets your views heard without escalating conflict. Heated discussions tend to start with accusations: "You did this!" Once someone feels blamed, they may escalate the tension: "No! You did that!" It pushes them to hold rigidly in their position. In sharp contrast, the I statement draws out empathy. When you lead with "I felt ___," or "I experienced ___," you activate someone's compassion. It often leads to conversations starting with an apology, "I'm sorry you felt that way; it wasn't my intention. I meant to ___."

Focus on the current issue

It is so easy to bring up past frustrations, especially if whatever troubles you feels like a pattern. This forces people to become defensive and can overwhelm them with the feeling that change is pointless or even impossible. You never want to suggest a behavior is "just the way you are," because that means there is no reason to even attempt the hard work of change. We can't alter the past, so don't revisit it.

Never belittle a feeling

It's common to comfort an upset person with a statement such as, "Don't worry about it," or "This is not that big a deal." These well-intentioned attempts at reassurance can backfire because they can feel belittling or minimizing. Instead say, "I hear how important this feels to you." Reinforce that you know they'll get through this challenge, and you'll be there as support.

Feelings are earned

In reliable relationships, people understand that feelings have a root cause. Even if an emotion is destructive to someone's well-being or undermining their progress, the feeling itself is never wrong because it is usually rooted in something the person experienced. Never lead with anything that implies, "You shouldn't be feeling _____." Start with something like, "I hear that you are feeling _____," or "I appreciate your trusting me enough to share your feelings." Productive conversations are started when thoughts and feelings are on the table.

Avoid saying "I understand"

When someone is upset, they will often respond with frustration to a person trying to express empathy who says, "I understand." They'll say, "How could you understand? You haven't been through this!" Instead, say, "Help me understand," or "I see you're hurting; tell me what you're feeling." Or "I can't imagine all that is going on. I'm here to listen. Tell me what I need to know to best support you."

A Path to Regain Trust

If our homes are to be reliable places where we can heal, we must never frame trust as broken. It can only be strained, leaving recovery always possible. We've considered communication pearls to lay the groundwork for productive and meaningful discussions. Now, let's consider a step-wise path to rebuilding trust. I carefully chose the word "path" rather than "plan." This is a journey, not an event that will meet with instant success.

Before you embark on this journey, have some concrete actions or strategies in mind you believe could improve matters. This prepares you for when an engaged partner in the discussion asks, "How?" to a general statement like, "Trust will need to be earned." Be ready with an answer, but invite them to offer their own solutions: "What do you think could work?" If their input is included, they'll more likely lean into the strategy.

Don't suggest everything will be solved easily. People should know hard work is both inevitable and worthwhile. If people go into any process of change believing it will come easily, they'll too quickly become demoralized by inevitable setbacks. Underscore that this is a journey by ending your first discussion with, "I feel a bit better. Why don't we talk about this again in 2 days?"

Here is a general strategy to follow.

1. With as little judgment as possible, state clearly why trust has been strained.
2. Explicitly state that trust can be re-earned and that you want to return to your most functional relationship.
3. Reinforce that you know who they really are, and all that you want is for them to return to their best self. (See the next chapter.)
4. Come up with a plan for how trust will be restored. Emphasize that it will be earned a step at a time.
5. Make it clear that you will monitor progress. Commit to watching more closely. Not because you don't trust. Not because you're trying to control. But because you care that much about your relationship being fully restored. If you are rebuilding trust with your child, add that you must monitor behavior because it is your role to guide them to be safe

and responsible. If this process is between you and a spouse, partner, or close relative, reinforce that regular check-ins on progress ensure you are both living up to your commitments to one another.

6. Come up with an action plan that has a clear first step. Tip: Make this first step attainable. When people achieve success in early attempts at change, they gain motivation to take the next, somewhat more difficult steps.

7. Agree to meet again shortly to discuss progress.

Put all of this in writing. Don't publicly display the agreement because you don't need a visible reminder of the tension. Remember also that children and teens resent public embarrassment and become angry if others learn of their problems. Having it in writing can prevent disagreements and serve as a starting point for the next discussion.

Final Thought

On the other side of any crisis can be a stronger relationship with a person who has once more learned the security you offer. Your reliable presence might be precisely what is needed for them to draw the strength to restore your relationship, recover from a challenge, or correct their behavior.

Resources

The Center for Parent and Teen Communication offers materials written by young people to help other youth understand their parents' viewpoint and how to effectively communicate with them.
https://parentandteen.com/category/talking-with-parents

It also includes teen-recommended strategies to rebuild trust with parents after relationship challenges or behavioral risk-taking.
https://parentandteen.com/category/for-teens/rebuilding-trust

CHAPTER 33

Riding the Waves by Seeing All That Is Good

This book, and my entire professional career is rooted in a strength-based approach. It is deeply protective to people to be seen as they deserve to be seen, as they really are, and not based on a behavior they might display in the moment or how they might perform. It makes humans feel valued. Known.

Parents viewing their children through a strength-based lens offers lifelong protection. As children journey through their lives even into the elder years, we want them to see themselves as worthy of healthy relationships and deserving of good things. But too many people don't feel as though they belong; in fact, they may live in fear of rejection. When a child knows that the person who knows them the most, inclusive of their challenges and their strengths, accepts them fully and chooses to love them unwaveringly, they will more likely see themselves as worthy of love. That's how much you matter. That's how much your being deeply intentional in seeing the best in your child may confer lifelong protection.

Seeing all that is good and right in your child makes a difference every day. But it will make the biggest difference when they are not displaying their best selves and you refuse to waver in seeing who they really are. Your child will feel most secure in this approach and will likely carry it forth into their own future relationships, if they see this approach taken in all relationships in your home . . . even in how you choose to see yourself.

Preparing for Adolescence

As your child stretches their wings into new territory, it's possible that not every decision will be wise or behavior reflective of their best self. It is during these more difficult moments that your strength-based approach will be critical in keeping your child grounded.

Shaping Your Lifelong Bond

Life becomes so full of contradictions. As adults, we must wear many hats to function, and even the most responsible person needs an occasional reminder of who they really are. You'll be the source of light that knows their core values and their essential character strengths. Similarly, as you age and your adult child may care for you, they'll remember how reliable you were when the rest of the world felt uncertain.

Remain a Source of Light They Can Seek Out

You see your child as no one else can. You know all their goodness and imagine all their potential. What else could possibly be a better source of light for a developing human than to be seen in this way? It's so much more than loving your child. It is about intentionally noticing their strengths. It's pretty easy to notice our children's strengths when they're being adorable. But remember, our deepest strengths may be revealed in the tougher moments. It's more than noticing when our children display resilience or remarkable compassion in these times. It's also that their deepest struggles may stem from their greatest strengths. For example, a child might experience social problems in school precisely because they stand by other children who are bullied or not accepted by most peers. Strategies to recognize and build on existing strengths were discussed more in depth in Chapter 7.

Whenever they need a safe and secure return

"... a safe and secure return." Return from where? To where should they return? In simplest terms, they should return to their best selves when they have strayed. When people do not live up to their potential or to their values, they don't feel good about themselves. People around them don't give them affirming messages; rather, they negatively react to their current behavior.

Sometimes we may not know who we are ourselves. We dwell in remorse or shame and struggle to imagine returning to a positive self-image. Humans need that North Star to remind them of who they are, to remember their potential, and to draw motivation to course correct when necessary. When you raise your children through a strength-based approach, your knowledge of who they are can always remain their North Star. You are the reminder of the source of light to which they want to return—their best, authentic self.

There is an added strategic reason to take a strength-based approach. It can prevent people from straying into unpleasant or dangerous territory in the first place. Children and teens are attention seekers. More than anything they want attention from their parents. They quickly learn what behaviors draw the most attention. All parents respond most emphatically to negative behavior and, unfortunately, that reinforces for young people that they draw attention with problematic behaviors. We provide a critical counterbalance when we notice and give attention to behaviors that demonstrate their essential goodness.

Love, respect, and caring as a framework for supportive change

I'd like to share an approach I teach professionals that respectfully engages young people who need to return to healthier, wiser behaviors. It invites people to problem-solve as experts on themselves, while clearly understanding 2 essential points.

- Our desire to correct them comes from a place of caring rooted in an understanding of their strengths.
- We are a guide who will remain involved and set protective rules.

I describe this as the "heart-belly-head-hands" approach. Even though the conversation should flow smoothly and does not explicitly mention each step, the framing reminds us to include each point. The heart message comes first because it underscores that our concern is rooted in caring and enables us to recount the precise reasons why they are deserving of, or have earned, our caring. The belly message describes our worry. This makes sense because our gut is often what signals us that we are worried. A gut instinct can even signal danger and the need for a course correction. Your head is where problems are solved. And your hands represent your unwavering presence and you reaching out to offer your support. When you follow this heart-belly-head-hands approach, you are implementing the best of balanced parenting—setting clear rules while expressing your caring.

- **Heart:** Share how deeply you care about your child. Make it clear that your caring is rooted in the special things you know about them. Name them.

  Breathe: Take a deep breath and pause to gather your thoughts. This shows that you are reflecting before you share. It models how we calm and collect ourselves.
- **Belly:** Explain precisely why you are worried. You worry that some of their choices may undermine the possibilities life holds for them or may interfere with others recognizing and supporting your child's potential.
- **Head:** In recognition of your child as the expert in their own life, invite them to consider a solution. Stay calm to enable them to engage their thoughtfulness. Share your thoughts and invite their comments. Brainstorm and arrive at a solution together.
- **Hands:** Tell your child you intend to support them and set the rules that will protect them. Ask their view of how you can best be supportive to them. Tell them that you might not have all the answers, but you guarantee your loving and guiding presence in their journey. Explore whether a professional could support their healing journey as well. (Refer to Chapter 22.)

If it's feeling hard to recall existing strengths

Being a parent does not relieve you of your human emotions. Amid a crisis, you might be so mired in anger or disappointment that accessing all your positive feelings about your child may be difficult. Give yourself a break. Take a look at past photos, recall joyful times, and fall in love again. Ask their teachers or friends' parents for their thoughts. It is likely they are seeing who your child really is despite the behavior you might be experiencing at home.

Say This (to your child)	Not That
These mistakes do not define you or make me love you even the slightest bit less. They just remind me that I should hold a mirror up to you more often so you can see what I see.	You are a real disappointment. You are not coming even close to your potential.
You are the same person you've always been. When I think of you, I think of _____.	You've really changed, haven't you? I remember when _____.
I hear how angry you are. You are so caring that you get easily frustrated.	You have a real anger problem.
It is not acceptable that you do _____. It is not consistent with your values.	No.

Humans Need to Be Seen Through a Positive Light

A strength-based approach benefits us all. As a family relationship is challenged, we hope to return your family to its best light. It was never a flawless family, because such a family doesn't exist. It is possible that the biggest stressors in your household exist between the adults. Each of your family members can grow and do so best when viewed through a positive lens. Members of your household can commit to doing better but through the same kind of mutual support that we give more generously and easily to children. This is what contributes to peace in our home, which we hope will make it a place your child will always return to for security. And in which the adults will thrive together even after the children have launched.

Say This (about another family member)	Not That
They care so much about you that their mood is affected deeply when they worry about you.	Just ignore them, they're having a bad day.
They are so sensitive that sometimes they need alone time to collect their feelings or sort out their thoughts. I am so glad I chose to share my life with someone so full of feelings. We all benefit from their sensitivity.	Give them space. They just need to settle themselves. (Note: There is nothing wrong with suggesting a person needs space. We all do sometimes. But when said with a tone that suggests, "They just need to settle," it implies their thoughts or feelings are out of control, rather than rooted in strengths they possess.)

You too . . .

Parents are often toughest on themselves in the moments when they are most deserving of grace. Precisely when our children are struggling and our stability and modeling of self-compassion are needed the most, we come down hard on ourselves. Your child may be struggling, but that doesn't mean you've messed up. It does mean that you're needed as part of the solution.

You're being watched. Model how you handle stress. Model that you are compassionate with yourself and forgiving even of mistakes. Even in the context of human errors, you remain good to your core and deeply committed to parenting. Consider what you are doing right as a parent and remember your own existing strengths. I don't know you, but I do know you are a committed parent, because you wouldn't be holding this book in your hand if you weren't trying to get this right.

And one more thought. You are so much more than a parent. Think about all the other gifts you bring to the world. Sit with those thoughts. Of course, you deserve growth. We all do. The respect for yourself and your commitment to continued self-improvement will serve as the best model of how your child sees you.

CHAPTER 34

Getting to the Goal:
Lifelong *Inter*dependence and
Mutual Support

We belong to each other. We thrive when we recognize that. Reliability is about being predictably present. We thrive when we rely on each other. We do so comfortably when our support is mutual. "Today, I will borrow your strength and wisdom. Tomorrow, I will lend you mine."

When we focus on raising our developing children, we naturally prepare them to launch into independent lives. As we should. We want our children fully prepared to be able to navigate this complicated world independently. But an overfocus on independence is a departure from something intuitively understood by our ancestors: Humans exist best in supportive units—families and communities. Only a small portion of our lives is spent raising our children in our homes. But we never stop being a parent. And we never stop being someone's child. Our parents' wisdom resides in our bone marrow.

We thrive when we understand that each of us contributes to our families and communities. Children bring endless joy and a reminder of how we should appreciate our surroundings, because miracles exist everywhere. Adolescents bring a questioning attitude and the potential for innovation and positive change. Adults perform the work of society and ensure the children are protected and that our basic needs are met. Elders share wisdom and experience. People thrive when we know we matter to one another, across the generations.

So, as we raise our children to be independent, we mustn't confuse that with the expectation that they will navigate the world alone. We want them endowed with the skills and confidence to handle life's complexities, but also with the deep-seated knowledge that they will succeed best when they choose *inter*dependence.

Preparing for Adolescence

The secret to your child appreciating your involvement in adolescence is that it feels like guidance, not control. It just so happens that when we get this right during the teen years, our adult children may be more likely to choose *inter*dependence with us.

Shaping Your Lifelong Bond

This chapter is intentionally the culmination of this book. There is no aspect of parenting a child more critical than raising them in a way that makes it more likely they will choose to form a lifelong bond. You should be the lighthouse that remains their enduring source of light and forever be seen as a reliable presence.

Influencing Our Children's Likelihood of Choosing Interdependence

The subtitle of this book gives away my intentions. Indeed, Lighthouse Parenting is more than just a strategy to apply balanced parenting, the approach proven to produce children with the best emotional, behavioral, and academic outcomes. Applying the principles of balanced parenting is a strategy for "Raising Your Child With Loving Guidance for a Lifelong Bond" because it strengthens families. If the subtitle didn't show all my cards, I underscored this point in every chapter with a thought about how each topic contributed to "Shaping Your Lifelong Bond." Much of this book promoted parenting practices that will make it more likely that your child will choose to be *inter*dependent with you over their lifetime. Let's highlight a few key points.

Parental love must be unconditional and unwavering. We love so that our children know they are worthy of being loved. This gift is so profound and authentically unconditional love so rare that the connection between people sharing this type of love is enduring.

We must know our child as few others could. People try on so many different hats in various settings that it is easy to lose our core identity. A parent best understands who their child is and has always been. Someone with this knowledge is irreplaceable.

We should enjoy each other. People need and deserve to enjoy their lives despite the hardships likely to be endured. Create good lasting memories. Enjoy the little things life offers. Create a habit of sharing those moments and both you and your child will want them to continue.

We must be warm, but not act as friends. You will likely grow into a sort of friendship with your adult child. But your child needs your unwavering presence even when you don't like what they are doing. Friendships come and go in childhood. Children may feel forced to do what it takes to fit in with friends. Your relationship as a parent is vitally needed precisely because it is stronger and more secure than any friendship.

We should value how our children add to our lives. If our children feel like a burden or a constant source of stress, they'll be driven to relieve you of that perceived burden. Instead, let your child know all the ways they add value to your life.

We should help our child know that they matter and can contribute to others' lives. Knowing that you matter can drive people to positive behaviors. And they matter to you. Let them know in childhood so they'll always know their presence contributes to your life.

We should see children as the experts in their own lives. Helping them realize that you see them as best understanding their own lives takes away the fear that their thoughts, feelings, or behaviors will be brushed aside.

We should guide, not dictate. Guides are welcome in our lives. Nobody of any age likes to be told what to do. Your child will forever remember whether their own views were heard.

We should honor their growing independence. When parents support their children's inevitable march toward independence, children learn they are allowed to grow. Once they can confidently stand on their own, they will choose to have someone standing alongside them. When parents thwart independence, people learn to go it alone.

We should avoid installing control buttons. Adults need to be respected to make decisions on their own; otherwise, they do not let others nearby. When parents install control buttons in their children, by telling them what to do and disrupting developing independence, adult children will limit their presence and choose not to share information with them.

We should support the growth that comes from recovery after temporary failures. Life is full of failures. When parents see failure as disastrous or to be avoided at all costs, adult children may learn to share only their successes and therefore withhold much of their lives from their parents. When failure is seen as a learning and growing opportunity, less of our real lives has to be hidden.

We should express concerns about anything that compromises our child's safety. It is our job to prevent irreparable harm. Our children really appreciate feeling protected. Our adult children will likely want to continue to include people in their life that are watching out for their well-being.

It's Only Beginning

When I have the privilege of giving a community talk, I have come to expect a few parents will approach me with a sense of urgency. They talk to me with a clear lump building in their throat. These parents tend to react with a sense of mourning or a foreboding feeling about 3 key points in development.

- The "end" of childhood
- The approach of the teen years
- The looming departure of their adolescent children from their homes

I try to explain that their sense of urgency, while understandable, is not merited. I underscore that our relationships with our children will continue for decades and that each phase brings opportunities for growth and strengthened relationships. Let's consider each of these concerns.

The "end" of childhood. There is a joy and innocence of childhood. And you may miss it when it's gone, but it will be replaced by new experiences that will be magical to witness. Don't make your child grow up too soon. But as they grow into adults never let them let go of their playfulness or the awe they experience by their surroundings. Those elements of childhood should be timeless.

The approach of the teen years. Some people fear adolescence. This is largely because people don't understand it. While this developmental stage can bring challenges, it can also be an inspirational time in which you celebrate the adult coming into view. Don't worry, I've got your back with my book *Congrats—You're Having a Teen! Strengthen Your Family and Raise a Good Person.* (You caught me, the subtitle gives away my intention again.) You'll be well prepared with this guide.

The looming departure of their adolescent children from their homes. People worry their job is done when their child leaves home or that their influence will wane. If you think of child-rearing as a job, your job becomes part time and often virtual after your child leaves home. But your role in each other's lives has not diminished. Important tip: Reject the term "empty nest." It is an awful concept that will leave you feeling barren and lonely at best. Words matter. They set the tone for how we view and experience something. Instead, look forward to your child being "in flight." Celebrate that they are comfortable soaring on their own. Be confident they will choose to return to your nest for landings.

Closure

If I made this parenting thing sound easy, then I failed you. I'm sorry. If I made it sound like hard work that is vital to your well-being and well worth the investment, then I've hit the mark. When you close this book, please let these words linger: **You must first care for yourself before you can care for others.** Self-care is necessary for your own well-being, but it is also a strategic act of effective parenting because you model the adult your child will become. I know I say that often, but you deserve to hear it.

As I write the closing words of this book, I just returned home from dinner with both my 28-year-old daughters. We laughed a lot. Among other things, they teased me for the inevitability of me staining my clothes. Tonight, it was soy sauce on my new (well, thrifted) sweater. I offered some wisdom. I received better advice than I offered. We shared a piece of chocolate cake honestly larger than half my head. (Don't worry, it was the good-for-you kind because it also had a sliced strawberry on it.) They're my best friends. If I had said that when they were 16, it wouldn't have been what they needed. They needed a parent then. Now it feels so right to be both a parent and a friend.

Breathe. Your relationship with your children is just beginning.

Index